NEW PERSPECTIVES IN LUNG CANCER

NEW PERSPECTIVES IN LUNG CANCER

Edited by
NICK THATCHER
Cancer Research Campaign Department of Medical Oncology,
Christie Hospital NHS Trust and Wythenshawe Hospital,
Manchester

and

STEPHEN SPIRO
Departments of General and Thoracic Medicine,
University College Hospital and Royal Brompton National Heart
and Lung Hospitals, London

Published by the BMJ Publishing Group
Tavistock Square, London WC1H 9JR

First published 1994

British Library Cataloguing in Publication Data

A catalogue record for this book is available
from the British Library

ISBN 0–7279–0786–7

Chapters 3, 4, 5, 8, and 9 are revised versions of articles
from *Thorax*

The cover illustration comprises a radiograph showing a bronchoscope
inserted into a chest. This was provided by M Muers.

Typeset, printed and bound in Great Britain by
Latimer Trend & Company Ltd, Plymouth

Contents

Page

Preface

1 Tobacco and lung cancer   1
   ANNE CHARLTON, *director, Cancer Research Campaign*
   Education and Child Studies Research Group,
   Department of Public Health and Epidemiology,
   Stopford Building, University of Manchester

2 Genetic changes in lung cancer   19
   ANTHONY BENCH, *research student*
   PAMELA RABBITTS, *senior scientist, Medical Research*
   Council, Clinical Oncology and Radiotherapeutics Unit,
   Hills Road, Cambridge

3 Neuroendocrine differentiation on lung tumours   30
   MARY N SHEPPARD, *consultant, Department of Lung*
   Pathology, National Heart and Lung Institute, Royal
   Brompton National Heart and Lung Hospital, London

4 Growth factors and lung cancer   51
   PENELLA J WOLL, *lecturer in medical oncology, Cancer*
   Research Campaign Department of Medical Oncology,
   Christie Hospital NHS Trust, Manchester

5 The antigens of lung cancer   68
   ROBERT L SOUHAMI, *professor, Department of*
   Oncology, Courtauld Institute of Biochemistry, London

6 How much investigation?   77
   MARTIN F MUERS, *consultant, Regional Cardiothoracic*
   Unit, Killingbeck Hospital, Leeds

7 Recent clinical trials in advanced lung cancer 105
DAVID J GIRLING, *senior scientist, MRC Cancer Trials
Office, 1 Brooklands Avenue, Cambridge*
NICHOLAS THATCHER, *reader in medical oncology,
Cancer Research Campaign Department of Medical
Oncology, Christie Hospital NHS Trust and
Wythenshawe Hospital, Manchester*

8 Haematopoietic growth factors and lung cancer
treatment 120
NICHOLAS THATCHER, *reader in medical oncology,
Cancer Research Campaign Department of Medical
Oncology, Christie Hospital NHS Trust and
Wythenshawe Hospital, Manchester*
HEATHER ANDERSON, *consultant, Cancer Research
Campaign Department of Medical Oncology,
Wythenshawe Hospital, Manchester, and Christie
Hospital NHS Trust, Manchester*

9 New drugs in lung cancer 143
DENIS C TALBOT, *consultant, University of Oxford
ICRF Clinical Oncology Unit, Churchill Hospital,
Headington, Oxford*
IAN E SMITH, *consultant medical oncologist,
Department of Medicine, Royal Marsden Hospital,
Sutton, Surrey*

10 Quality of Life 161
PENELOPE HOPWOOD, *honorary consultant psychiatrist,
Cancer Research Campaign Psychological Medicine
Group, Stanley House, Christie Hospital NHS Trust,
Manchester*
ANN CULL, *consultant clinical psychologist, ICRF
Medical Oncology Unit, Western General Hospital,
Edinburgh*

11 Patient benefit in clinical trials 177
MAURICE L SLEVIN, *consultant, Department of Medical
Oncology, St Bartholomew's Hospital, West Smithfield,
London*
JEAN MOSSMAN, *Secretary, United Kingdom
Co-ordinating Committee on Cancer Research, London*

Index 185

Preface

Interest in lung cancer has gripped the imagination over the past few years, and *New Perspectives in Lung Cancer* addresses the important advances in understanding of the biology of lung cancer and particular management issues.

Genetic studies and new histological techniques for identifying neuroendocrine features of lung tumours have provided important new information. Growth regulation and specific cellular antigens that could lead to targeted therapy are also discussed. Another chapter emphasises the importance of avoiding unnecessary investigations.

Other aspects of treatment are discussed within the context of clinical trials, particularly from large multicentre groups. Examples are given of the effect of these trials in determining future clinical management and the optimal use of scarce resources. New aspects of treatment, including the reduction in myelosuppression from chemotherapy with haematopoietic growth factors and new chemotherapy drugs in lung cancer, indicate ways of improving treatment in the future.

Two other important issues are addressed. Firstly, tobacco, which has been identified as a particular problem in young schoolchildren; indeed 10% of schoolchildren now smoke rather than the 8% quoted in *The Health of the Nation* in July 1992. Secondly, the chapter on patients' quality of life highlights the fact that medical assumptions can be incorrect—more treatment can be associated with a better quality of life. How to measure quality of life and the importance of doing so are discussed, as is the potential benefit to patients treated within a clinical trial context.

The present lively interest in lung cancer will assist in developing new strategies for prevention and treatment not only in this common cancer but also in other types of cancer, thereby overcoming the climate of pessimism which is a major obstacle to progress.

N Thatcher
S Spiro
December 1993

1 Tobacco and lung cancer

ANNE CHARLTON

Lung cancer is a disease which is, at present, almost always fatal; it could be almost entirely prevented, but is not.

About 158 000 new patients are registered with lung cancer in the European Community each year,[1] where it is the commonest cancer in men, making up over 20% of all new cancer cases anually. The picture is similar in the United States: the surgeon general's report 1992 indicates that 133 700 deaths from lung cancer occur annually in North America.

About 40 000 new patients are registered in the United Kingdom each year,[1] where a quarter of the total number of deaths from cancer are caused by lung cancer.

For some time now, lung cancer has been the most common cause of cancer death among men and the second for women. Since 1984, however, deaths from lung cancer have exceeded those from breast cancer among women in Scotland and in some parts of northern England, and lung cancer is set to overtake breast cancer as the major cancer killer of women in other areas.

The incidence of lung cancer has not always been this high. In 1849 John Hughes Bennett in Edinburgh wrote, "This is the only case of cancer of the lung which I have ever met with; so I presume the disease rarely attacks this organ in Scotland."[2] This is a particularly ironic statement in view of current lung cancer incidence in Scotland. Others, such as Walshe[3] in 1843 felt that, "It is important for the practitioner to be aware that cancer of the lung is far from being an affection of such uncommon occurrence as is generally supposed." Kilgour also urged caution in 1850 when he said that intrathoracic cancer was "a disease which, I am satisfied,

1

is more common than it is supposed to be by the profession, and which, unless a careful examination be made, both of the history of the case, and of the physical signs attending it, is very apt to be mistaken for some other complaint".[4]

Osler (1892) showed the increased risk of lung cancer in cobalt miners in Schneeberg[5]; Loomis (1875)[6] found that the disease was more common in men than in women and that the main incidence was between the ages of 40 and 60 years, and Hartshorne (1885)[7] and Loomis both supported the idea of some hereditary factor being involved. In 1885 Fitz[8] suggested that in the cause of lung cancer "the existence of an irritant of some sort seems possible". If tobacco smoking had been shown then to be the major cause of lung cancer that we now know it to be, how different might be the present situation.

These quotations were collected into a review of lung cancer in the nineteenth century by Onuigbo in 1959.[9] He ends his review by drawing the reader's attention to the lack of success obtained by any treatment methods for lung cancer in the nineteenth century and the deep despondency of the physicians at that time. For example, Salter (1869)[10] said in his clinical lectures, "With regard to *treatment*, gentlemen, I need not tell you that I have *nothing* to tell you". He expressed his pessimism as, "doubt if we can in such a case put off the final catastrophe for a single hour". Onuigbo, in his intriguing review, says, "Today, we do look forward to some success after surgery. The gloom of yesteryear is being lifted." The survival rate is still low, however, and even early treatment seems to have relatively little success.

About the time that Onuigbo was writing, the cause of most lung cancer had recently been identified. Cigarette smoking was shown by Doll and Hill in the United Kingdom[11-13] and by Hammond and Horn in the United States of America[14 15] to be significantly associated with lung cancer. The major cause had been found; the disease could be almost entirely prevented; but the subsequent story is a strange and illogical one.

Lung cancer trends

Mortality rates have been recorded since the beginning of the twentieth century. At that time, fewer than 10 deaths per 100 000 men were due to lung cancer. Although this may be slightly lower than the true rate, due to relatively poor diagnosis, it was certainly

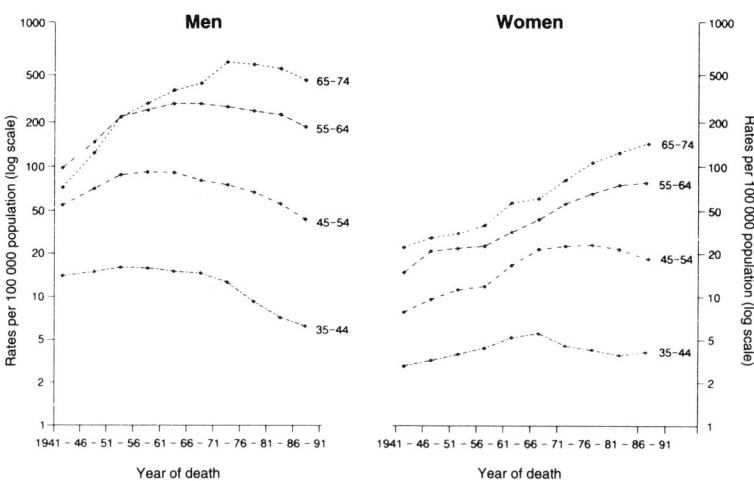

Mortality time trends

England & Wales 1941-1990

Figure 1   Lung cancer mortality in England and Wales.

Figure reproduced from Cancer Research Campaign Factsheet II:1 *Lung Cancer and Smoking—UK*. Cancer Research Campaign, London, 1992. Based on data from *Cancer Mortality, England and Wales 1911–1970*. SMPS No 29. OPCS Monitors DH1 80/3 and 82/2. London: OPLS, 1980, 1982. *Mortality Statistics: cause. England and Wales*. DH2 Nos 8–17. London: HMSO.

well below that of the 1950s when lung cancer mortality among men had risen to 60 per 100 000 and to over 100 per 100 000 men by the 1980s. Since then, lung cancer mortality among men has declined.[16] For women, mortality rates in the older age groups are still rising.

It is now known that most deaths from lung cancer are caused by tobacco smoke, and the pattern of lung cancer incidence follows that of the prevalence and consumption of cigarettes (figures 1 and 2). The main carcinogenic agent or agents are thought to be in the tar contained in the cigarette smoke which settles in the trachea, bronchi, and lungs. As with most carcinogens, it is some years before lesions become apparent. This is one of the main problems in convincing governments in developing countries, where the cigarette habit is relatively new and is being aggressively marketed by the tobacco industry, that health problems will arise. They do not see a major health problem related to smoking at present and therefore are sometimes unwilling to take action to prevent something in the future which is, as yet, invisible. Financially it would

3

Percentage of population who smoke

Great Britain 1948–1987 — men and women aged 16 and over

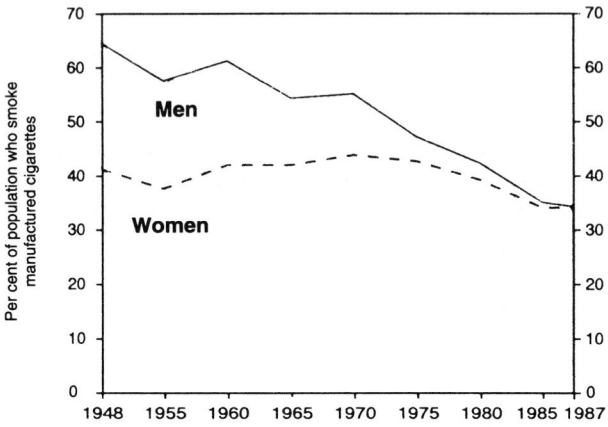

Figure 2   Smoking prevalence in adults.

Figure reproduced from Cancer Research Campaign Factsheet II:2 *Lung Cancer and Smoking—UK*. Cancer Research Campaign, London, 1992.
Data from *UK Smoking Statistics*. Second Edition. Oxford: Oxford University Press, 1991, based on Tobacco Advisory Council research.[20][21]

be worth their while: a study in Northern Ireland in 1986 showed that expenditure in health care related to tobacco alone amounted to £10 360 000 in 1984.[17]

Trends in smoking

In the nineteenth century men usually smoked pipes or cigars, but with the development of cigarette manufacturing machinery, cigarettes quickly took over as the main method of smoking early in the twentieth century. Until then many working men would not have been habitual smokers because clay pipes required a lot of lighting, tamping, and careful handling; cigarettes could be smoked easily at any time and carried around in pockets. Inhalation from cigarettes was also more frequent (and still is) than it was from pipes and cigars. Men's cigarette consumption of manufactured cigarettes rose from 800 a person in 1905 to 4420 per person in 1945, fell sharply after the war to 3320 in 1949, after which it rose again to 4030 in 1960.[18] The publication of the first report on smoking by the Royal College of Physicians in 1962[19] might have

4

had an effect in that men's cigarette consumption then began a general downward trend to reach 2380 in 1985.

Women have shown a different pattern of consumption. Starting in 1921, with 13 cigarettes a person, the trend was steadily upward for the next 50 years, reaching 1250 in 1945, and peaking at 2630 in 1974. Since then, women's cigarette consumption has also fallen, but more slowly than that of men, being 1930 a person in 1985.

Consumption and prevalence are to some extent related. Several long term surveys have monitored prevalence.[20-22] Their findings are slightly different due to methodology and wording of questions, but the salient points are the same. The Tobacco Advisory Council's (TAC) studies[20 21] have been running the longest and their findings are those which are shown in figure 2. The General Household Surveys[22] have included questions on smoking since 1972 and their findings are largely similar to those of TAC—namely, that the prevalence of cigarette smoking among men has decreased from 52% in 1972 to 31% in 1990; smoking prevalence among women has fallen from 41% in 1972 to 29% in 1990.

Within these overall statistics are concealed two important factors which will, in the future, be reflected in the pattern of lung cancer cases. These are: (1) that smoking prevalence among young women under 25 has increased in recent years; and (2) that most of the cigarette smokers are in the less affluent socioeconomic status groups.[21] Figure 3 shows how, although smoking prevalence in the more affluent socioeconomic groups has fallen sharply, the decrease in the less affluent groups is much less noticeable. The risk of an unskilled working man dying of lung cancer is three times that of a professional man, and smoking is clearly a major contributor to this difference.

It is only comparatively recently that data on prevalence of smoking have been collected from children and young people.[23-27] A national survey which was conducted in 1966 excluded girls, on the basis that they did not smoke, and focused on boys,[28] although some regional surveys at the same time found regular smoking to be as high as 20% in 14 and 15 year old girls. At that stage the smoking prevalence was 4% for 11 and 12 year old boys and 27% for 14 and 15 year olds. Until 1982 no further national surveys were carried out in secondary schools, but then regular surveys to be carried out every two years were instituted by the Department of Health. Carried out by the Social Surveys Division of the Office of Population Censuses and Surveys, the findings of these surveys

5

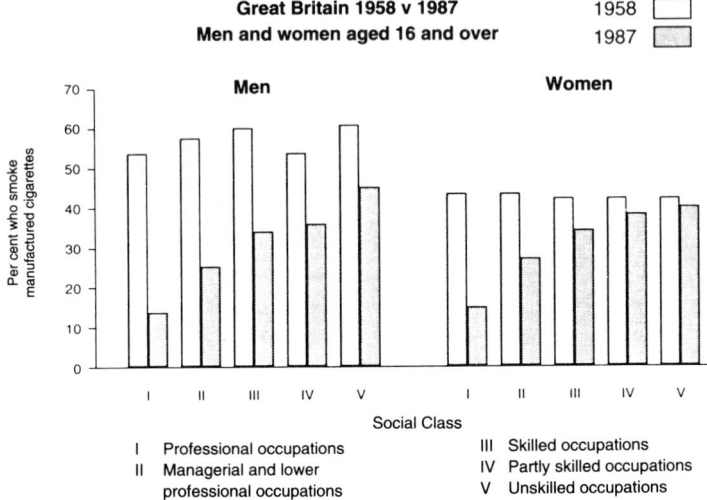

Percentage who smoke by social class

Figure 3   Changes in smoking prevalence related to socioeconomic status.

Figure reproduced from Cancer Research Campaign Factsheet II:3 *Lung Cancer and Smoking—UK*. Cancer Research Campaign, London, 1992.
Data from *UK Smoking Statistics*. Second Edition. Oxford: Oxford University Press, 1991, based on Tobacco Advisory Council research.

are shown in the table. The most alarming features are the high prevalence among girls in their early teens, relative to that of boys, and the fact that a quarter of the 15 year olds are smoking during their last year at school. Most smokers start the habit before they reach the age of 19 years, so young people are of particular relevance if lung cancer is to be prevented, especially in view of the powerfully addictive nature of the nicotine in the tobacco smoke.

The risk of lung cancer is related to the length of time a person has been a regular smoker rather than to the amount smoked. For example, 20 cigarettes a day for 30 years produces a greater risk than 40 cigarettes a day for 15 years. Doll and Peto have shown how greatly the risk of lung cancer in later life is increased if a person starts regular smoking in their teens.[29][30]

Passive smoking

It is not only the smokers themselves who create a personal risk of lung cancer. There is now evidence that inhalation of other

6

TABLE I   Smoking behaviour of 11 to 15 year olds (per cent) by sex: England 1982 to 1990

	1982	1984	1986	1988	1990
Boys					
Regular smoker	11	13	7	7	9
Occasional smoker	7	9	5	5	6
Used to smoke	11	11	10	8	7
Tried smoking	26	24	23	23	22
Never smoked	45	44	55	58	56
Base (100%)	1460	1928	1676	1489	1643
Girls					
Regular smoker	11	13	12	9	11
Occasional smoker	9	9	5	5	6
Used to smoke	10	10	10	9	7
Tried smoking	22	22	19	19	18
Never smoked	49	46	53	59	58
Base (100%)	1514	1689	1508	1529	1478

Reproduced by permission from Lader D, Matheson J. *Smoking among Secondary School Children in 1990.* London: HMSO, 1991.

people's tobacco smoke on a long term basis is linked with an increased risk of lung cancer. Wives who live with husbands who smoke[31]; people who have been exposed to environmental tobacco smoke (ETS) in their homes both as children and as adults[32 33]; people who have been exposed to household ETS for 25 "smoker years" have all been found to have an increased risk of lung cancer.[34]

The reasons for smoking

The individual

In view of the widespread knowledge of the greatly increased risk of lung cancer and many other diseases associated with smoking, it seems strange that people continue with the habit. But, both the strong physiological addiction to the nicotine and the psychological aspects which accompany cigarette smoking make it very difficult for smokers, once "hooked", to give up. There are two sides to this question one of which lies with the individual and the other with society in general, but most specifically with the government (figure 4).

Taking the individual aspects first, these usually apply in youth when most smokers establish their habit.[35] First, parental influence

7

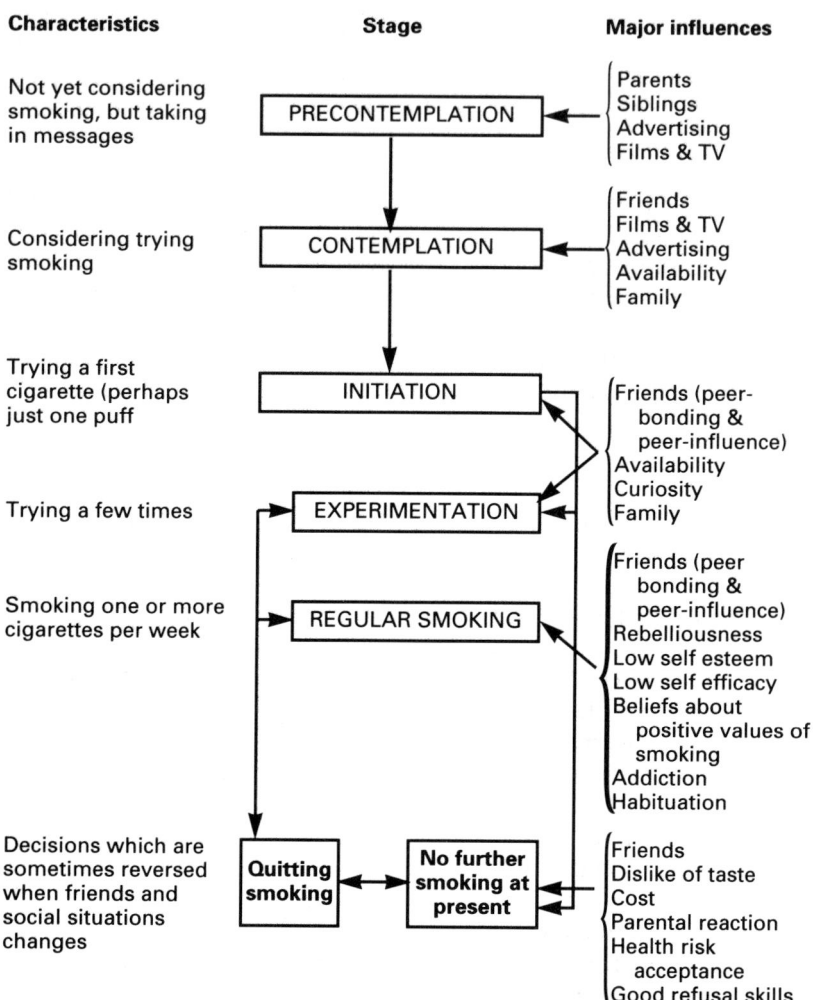

Figure 4   Stages in the development of smoking.

Reproduced from *Smoking and the Young*. London, Royal College of Physicians, 1992.

and example is the first influence young children meet. It is at home that their primary socialisation takes place. Children whose parents smoke are twice as likely to be smokers as those with non-smoking parents.[36] There are several possible reasons for this, one being the actual availability of cigarettes and the fact that cigarette smoking is seen as the norm. With regard to the first of these reasons, a major study showed that 1% of young smokers had tried at least a puff of a cigarette before they were 4 years old.[37] The smoking norm is established early and can be associated with security.

It is unrealistic to tackle the problem among children at school without providing them with back-up from adults. Once a child starts school, friends and peers become very important. The need to conform with the group can overtake parental influence. Peer bonding, where being or not being a smoker is one of the common factors in each group of friends, or peer pressure, where children who smoke intimidate others into taking up the habit both play a part.[38] Natural curiosity leads many children to try a first cigarette, but other factors influence their continuation with the habit. Many children try a first cigarette and, for whatever reason, decide not to try another. Other children persist with experimentation. It is certain that many young people are addicted quite early in their smoking history,[39] although most believe that it would be easy to stop and that they could do so whenever they want to.[40] This is clearly not the case as research has shown.[41] Many young people make repeated unsuccessful attempts at giving up and, although some are successful, it is often an uphill journey to reach this goal.

Other social factors influence young people's smoking habits: for example, role models and exemplars such as teachers, pop stars, sports personalities and older brothers and sisters. Teachers are seen as knowledgeable and, if they smoke, children and young people think it must be safe. Doctors and nurses who smoke are perceived as authorising the habit for children.

Over and above the influence of family, peers, and role models are the personal knowledge and beliefs held by the children themselves. Knowledge or admission of health risks seems to be a relatively unimportant factor in a child's decision to smoke[42] and can change with time as other influences, such as peer bonding, gain in importance. Such threats as lung cancer are not only far from perfectly understood, but they are also perceived as being too far ahead to be of any relevance whatsoever in a child's decision making process.[43] More immediate is what the young person thinks that smoking will do for him or her. The school age children most at risk of taking up smoking are often the rebellious or insecure ones.[44] Those who see themselves as underachievers in academic or behavioural terms, or who place little value on these generally accepted adult measures of personal worth have repeatedly been shown to be the most likely smokers. Weight control, confidence, calming nerves and most especially looking grown up and sophisticated are reasons for smoking which are most often believed by girls and are associated with their decision to smoke.[45] Girls with low self-esteem with regard to their physical appearance are most likely to fall for the image of cigarette smoking as being glamorous or "cool".

The process of taking up smoking is not necessarily a "once and for all" journey. Young people go in and out of smoking as they change friends, move from one school to another, or simply change their minds.

The state or government

Can the smoker really be blamed for his or her smoking habit? A long period of "victim blaming" ensued from 1962, when the first report of the Royal College of Physicians was published. The deeply rooted belief developed that once a person had been told about the health risks of smoking—especially that of lung cancer—they would and certainly *should* not smoke. But there are other issues besides that of health alone. The personal reasons mentioned earlier can far outweigh the risk of illness later in life. But perhaps most importantly, the serious health risks of cigarette smoking were now known, but marketing of tobacco continued as before. It would seem incredible to those physicians in the nineteenth century who despaired of treatment for lung cancer and desperately sought to identify the cause that so little has been done in the 40 years since the carcinogen was identified.

In fact, although smoking prevalence has declined, cigarettes are still marketed and advertised. How can an individual be blamed for accepting them? There are probably three main elements, apart from the fact that cigarettes are sold at all, which are crucial in the recruitment of new smokers and helping to ensure their maintenance of the habit.[46] These are availability, price, and advertising.

Cigarettes are widely available and, in the United Kingdom in 1989 50% of outlets sold cigarettes to children under the age of 16[47] which is against the law. Parents against Tobacco was formed and due to their efforts, the Protection of Young People (Tobacco) Bill increased fines for illegal sales and strengthened the legislation.[48] At least this action should reduce the availability of cigarettes to under 16s. It is hoped that it will be reflected in a reduction in smoking, but if tobacco can be sold only to people aged 16 and over, this may give the false impression that smoking is safe for adults and invest cigarettes with the glamour of "forbidden fruit". The tobacco industry, not surprisingly, supports this restriction.

The price of cigarettes has been shown in numerous studies in the United Kingdom[49] and the United States of America to be inversely related to demand. For every 1% increase in the real price of cigarettes there is roughly a 0·5% decrease in smoking.[50] The *real* price of cigarettes is calculated by relating the current price to the retail price index:

$$\text{Real price} = \frac{\text{current price}}{\text{retail price index}}$$

According to a study in the United States of America, adolescents are even more responsive to price than adults.[51] Low income groups are also particularly sensitive to price increases, and they reduce their smoking more as the real price of cigarettes rises and increase it as it falls.[52] It has been suggested that allowing the real price of cigarettes to fall between 1965 and 1980 in the United Kingdom could have contributed to the high prevalence of smoking in the lower socioeconomic groups. Most of the cost of a packet of cigarettes is tax and it therefore requires government action to increase this amount.

Problems arise with regard to an increase in tobacco taxes. A discussion of these issues was presented in a WHO publication in 1988.[50] The first is that it would reduce government revenue as sales would fall. This has been shown not to be the case; in fact increasing taxes increases government revenue while it decreases sales. The cost to the National Health Service would also be less. The second fear is that such price increases would be inflationary. If it is a tax increase alone, it takes money out of the economy and is therefore deflationary. If tobacco products are included in the retail price index, however, the result of the price increases could be fed into an inflationary spiral, if wages, pensions, etc, are linked to it. The Commission of the European Communities now publishes a retail price index which excludes tobacco and alcohol. Several countries have used tax increases to reduce smoking and have met with considerable success. Canada is one such country, but unfortunately this policy also seems to have led to a black market of lower priced cigarettes via the United States.[53]

11

How many people would support heroin advertising? Yet advertising of tobacco products continues. Tubes of paper containing dead leaves which can be lethal, the advertising suggests, are a symbol of elegance, confidence, toughness, friendship, sociability, or whatever a person wants them to mean. Whatever you want from life, smoking cigarettes will help you to attain it, say the advertisers. The voluntary agreement set out as the Cigarette Code in the British Code of Advertising Practice and monitored by the Committee for Monitoring Agreements on Tobacco Advertising and Sponsorship (COMATAS)—with equal numbers of representatives from the government and the tobacco industry in the United Kingdom—has eliminated the inclusion of young people, success, or sports prowess from the advertising of cigarettes in this country.[54] These restrictions are often circumvented by other means, especially sports sponsorship; even very young children are aware of cigarette advertising and understand its messages.[55] Awareness of at least one brand of cigarette was found to be one of the main predictors of smoking in the next few months for 12 and 13 year olds.[45] In the United States there is no such voluntary agreement, and imported magazines for young black people, which are widely read in Britain, contain exactly the type of advertisement from which the voluntary agreement should protect these people.

Cigarette advertising has been eliminated from British television since 1965 and advertising for cigars and tobacco ended in 1992. But sports sponsorship by tobacco companies related to cigarette brands continues. Children watch many of these sports.[56] A survey in late 1992 showed that, even at the age of 9 or 10 years, one in three children named at least one sport sponsored by a cigarette brand among their top television sports viewing. Research has shown increased awareness of the specific sponsoring cigarette brands following sponsored snooker championships.[57]

Even more subtle cigarette advertising appears in soap operas,[58] films, and in fashion photographs. Even children's films convey messages about smoking—for example, *Ghostbusters I* features main characters smoking and one of the *Superman* films includes a large delivery truck advertising a brand of cigarettes. The voluntary agreement ensures that no cigarette advertisements appear in magazines with 200 000 readers, one third of whom are aged between 16 and 24 years, but girls do not confine themselves to

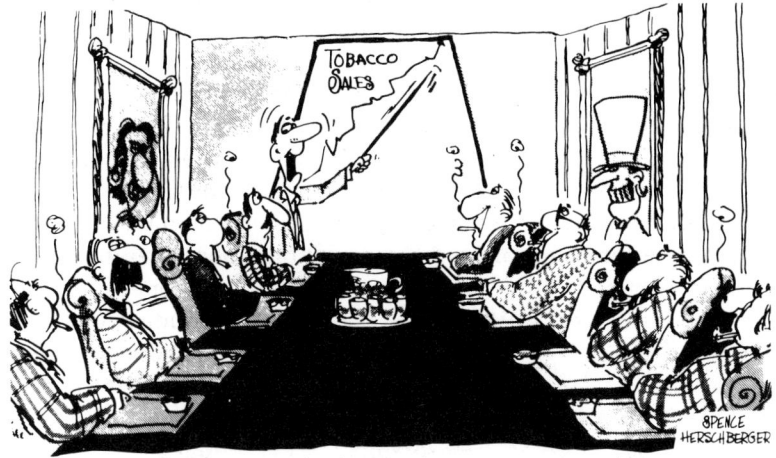

"At the same time, an unexplained percentage of our top customers continues to die, so advertising expenditures for new young customers are going to have to keep increasing."

Figure 5   The reason why the tobacco industry recruits young smokers.

Cartoon from *Smoking Is No Laughing Matter* by WR Spence, MD, and Vern Herschberger, 1987 Health EDCO.

these magazines. Cigarette advertisements and fashion models holding cigarettes or smoking can be seen in other magazines.

The tobacco industry loses over 300 adult customers in Britain every day from deaths related to smoking and more from others giving up smoking (figure 5). It therefore needs to attract the same number of young replacements every day. The clever, amusing, or visually beautiful cigarette advertisements are one way to attract young people's attention. Once hooked on nicotine, these young people provide continuing customers for the tobacco industry's profits.

The future?

Clearly, prevention is vastly better than cure for lung cancer and much more cost effective. There would be a tremendous reduction in the number of patients requiring treatment for lung cancer if cigarette smoking were to be prevented. So why does it not happen?

13

The trouble begins with the tobacco industry itself. A revealing statement was made by Dr Lionel Blackman, the director of research and development for British–American Tobacco Industries Ltd (BAT) in 1981.[59]

"Despite a never-ending stream of research on the possible health hazards of smoking, there is no proof of a cause-and-effect relationship between cigarette smoking and various alleged smoking diseases."[60]

It is clear that no amount of evidence will make producers of tobacco products admit to the harm their products are causing. Too much money is involved.

Since the early 1960s the government's approach has almost always been targeted to the individual, and almost all the finance and effort has been directed to children in school. First came the boring health lectures illustrated by black lungs in jars. This method proved largely ineffective, so psychological approaches were introduced instead. Fishbein's theory of reasoned action was tried, where the child was asked to weigh up his personal beliefs about being a non-smoker related to what other people would think of his decision;[61] Becker's Health Belief Model was applied in which the child works through four stages as follows[62]: Is this a serious health risk? Is it a risk to me personally? What will I lose by my choice? What will I gain by it? This process often fell at the second fence because the risk of lung cancer was neither understood nor seen as personal by the child. Decision making skills, peer led teaching, social influences, attempts to resist peer pressure and many other approaches have been tried. An excellent overview of the many models and theories which underpin health education was presented by Tones in 1990.[63] In the United States of America a valuable analysis was made of the various intervention programmes and their effects.[64] The conclusion was that it was possible to achieve a limited and perhaps short term effect on delaying the onset of smoking among young people. A set of indicators for planning school intervention programmes was developed and is very useful.[65]

In England in 1989 the government allocated a considerable amount of money to the Health Education Authority to reduce teenage smoking. Some excellent programmes have been developed and monitoring has been carried out every six months. The national surveys indicate, however, that there has been no significant change in smoking prevalence in secondary school children between 1982 and 1990. An evaluation of two of the most important programmes has shown that they do not produce the level of effect which was hoped for.[66] Perhaps it is too early to observe the effects of the programme, but it is also likely that the emphasis is misplaced. Whatever the health education methods, is it fair to place the entire onus of being a non-smoker on a child while the adult world continues to sell and advertise and smoke cigarettes? Giving talks in schools is not the answer.

Instead of tackling the problem from the bottom up and placing the responsibility firmly with the individual, a top-down approach is now essential. Government action is needed to ban advertising, to increase taxes on cigarettes, to ensure that whenever possible cigarette smoking is not portrayed as desirable, and to create no-smoking areas on public transport and other public areas. The ideal situation would be to ban all promotion of tobacco products. People should not have to make the decision as to whether or not they will use this lethal drug.

On 14 February 1990, tests in North Carolina found benzene concentrations of 12 to 20 parts per million, about four times the safe level, in bottled mineral water. Although United States authorities said that, "the chances of developing cancer as a result of drinking Perrier water (are) tiny; drinkers would need to consume half a litre a day for 30 years to be exposed to a million-to-one risk".[67] Nevertheless, by 15 February distributors in the United States, Canada, Japan, Germany, the Netherlands and Denmark stopped all sales of the product. The manufacturers, Perrier, immediately withdrew all supplies of the water worldwide. On the other hand, quite apart from its many other harmful contents, sidestream smoke contains more than 400 µg of benzene per cigarette, polluting one cubic metre of air in a public place with 20–317 µg[68]—far more than in the contaminated water—and yet the manufacturers actively *promote* it. Benzene is, of course, only one of numerous carcinogens found in tobacco smoke.

Lung cancer is a political disease. Powerful people see the threat to their personal profits as an obstacle to removing its cause. A steady and significant decrease in the number of cigarettes con-sumed could have a far greater effect on the Health of the Nation, one of whose targets is "To reduce the death rate for lung cancer by at least 30 per cent in men under 75 and 15 per cent in women under 75 by 2010."[69].

15

TOBACCO AND LUNG CANCER

1 Cancer Research Campaign. *Lung cancer and smoking: Factsheet II. Cancer in the European Community. Factsheet V.* London: Cancer Research Campaign, 1992.
2 Bennett JH. *On cancerous and cancroid growth.* Edinburgh: Sutherland and Knox, 1849;45.
3 Walshe WH. *The physical diagnosis of diseases of the lungs.* London: Taylor and Walton, 1843:285.
4 Kilgour A. Cases of cancer in the thorax. *Monthly Journal of Medical Science*, 1850;**10**:508–23.
5 Osler W. *The principles and practice of medicine.* London: Young J Pentland, 1892:556.
6 Loomis AL. *Lectures on the respiratory organs, heart and kidneys.* New York: William Wood and Co, 1875:118.
7 Hartshorne H. General etiology, medical diagnosis and prognosis. In: Pepper W, Starr L, eds. *A system of practical medicine: Vol 1 Pathology and general diseases.* London: Sampson Low, Marston, Searle and Rivington, 1885:129.
8 Fitz RH. General morbid processes; inflamation; thrombosis and embolism; effusions; degenerations; tuberculosis; morbid growths. In: Pepper W, Starr L, eds. *A system of practical medicine: Vol 1 Pathology and general diseases.* London: Sampson Low, Marston, Searle and Rivington, 1985:108.
9 Onuigbo WIB. Lung cancer in the nineteenth century. *Medical History.* 1959;**3**:69–77.
10 Salter H. Clinical lectures on diseases of the chest. Lecture 1: On primary cancer of the lung. *Lancet* 1869;ii:1–4.
11 Doll R, Hill AB. The study of the aetiology of carcinoma of the lung. *Br J Cancer* 1952;ii:1271–86.
12 Doll R, Hill AB. The mortality of doctors in relation to their smoking habits. A preliminary report. *Br Med J* 1954;i:1451–5.
13 Doll R, Hill AB. Lung cancer and other causes of death in relation to smoking. A second report on the mortality of British doctors. *Br Med J* 1956;ii:1071–81.
14 Hammond EC, Horn D. Smoking and death-rates—a report on forty-four months of follow-up of 187,783 men. I. Total mortality. *JAMA* 1958;**166**:1159–72.
15 Hammond EC, Horn D. Smoking and death rates—a report on forty-four months of follow-up of 187, 783 men. II. Deaths by cause. *JAMA* 1958;**166**:1294–308.
16 Royal College of Physicians of London. *Smoking or health.* Tunbridge Wells: Pitman Medical Publishing, 1977.
17 Ulster Cancer Foundation. The economic consequences of smoking in Northern Ireland: a cost benefit analysis of tobacco production and use in the province. Belfast: Ulster Cancer Foundation, 1986.
18 Wald N, Kiryluk S, Darby S, Doll R, Pike M, Peto R. *UK smoking statistics.* Oxford: Oxford University Press, 1988.
19 Royal College of Physicians of London. *Smoking and health. A report on smoking in relation to lung cancer and other diseases.* Tunbridge Wells: Pitman Medical Publishing, 1962.
20 Todd GF, ed. *Statistics of smoking in the United Kingdom (Research Paper 1).* First Edition. London: Tobacco Research Council, 1957.
21 Lee PN. *Statistics of smoking in the United Kingdom (Research paper 1).* Seventh Edition. London: Tobacco Research Council, 1976.
22 Office of Population Censuses and Surveys. Cigarette smoking 1972–1990. In: *General Household Survey*: OPCS Monitor SS91/3. London: OPCS 1991.
23 Dobbs J, Marsh A. *Smoking among secondary school children in 1982.* London: HMSO, 1983.
24 Dobbs J, Marsh A. *Smoking among secondary school children in 1984.* London: HMSO, 1985.
25 Goddard E, Ikin C. *Smoking among secondary school children in 1986.* London: HMSO, 1987.
26 Goddard E. *Smoking among secondary school children in 1988.* London: HMSO, 1989.
27 Lader D, Matheson J. *Smoking among secondary school children in 1990.* London: HMSO, 1991.
28 Bynner JM. *The young smoker.* London: HMSO, 1969.
29 Doll R, Peto R. *The causes of cancer.* Oxford: Oxford University Press, 1981.
30 Peto R. Influence of dose and duration of smoking on lung cancer rates. In: Zarridge DG, Peto R, eds. *Tobacco: a major international health hazard.* Lyon, France: International Agency for Research on Cancer, 1986:23–33.
31 Hirayama T. Non-smoking wives of heavy smokers have a higher risk of lung cancer. *Br Med J* 1981;**282**:183–5.

16

32 Correa P, Pickle LW, Fontham E, Lin Y, Haenszel W. Passive smoking and lung cancer. *Lancet* 1983;ii:595–7.
33 Sandler DP, Wilcox AJ, Everson RB. Cumulative effects of lifetime passive smoking on cancer risk. *Lancet* 1985;i:312–15.
34 Janerich DT, Thompson WD, Varela LR, *et al.* Lung cancer and exposure to tobacco smoke in the household. *N Engl J Med* 1990;323:632–6.
35 Royal College of Physicians of London. *Smoking and the young.* London: RCP, 1992.
36 Aaro LE, Hauknes A, Berglund E-L. Smoking among Norwegian schoolchildren 1975–1980. II The influence of the social environment. *Scand J Psychol* 1981;22:297–309.
37 Charlton A. The Brigantia Survey: a general review. *Public Education about Cancer* 1984;77:92–102.
38 Flay BR, d'Avernas JR, Best JA, Kersell MW, Ryan KB. Cigarette smoking: why young people do it and ways of preventing it. In: McGrath P, Firestone P, eds. *Pediatric and adolescent behavioral medicine.* New York: Springer-Verlag, 1983:132–83.
39 McNeill AD. The development of dependence on smoking in children. *Br J Addict* 1991;86:589–92.
40 Charlton A, Melia P, Moyer C. eds. *A manual on tobacco and young people for the Industrialised World.* Geneva: International Union Against Cancer, 1990.
41 Marsh A, Matheson J. *Smoking attitudes and behaviour.* London: HMSO, 1983.
42 Swan AV, Murray M, Jarrett L. *Smoking behaviour from pre-adolescent to young adulthood.* Aldershot: Avebury, 1991.
43 Bland JM, Bewley BR, Banks MH, Pollard V. Schoolchildren's beliefs about smoking and disease. *Health Ed J* 1975;34:71–8.
44 Stewart L, Livson N. Smoking and rebelliousness: a longitudinal study from childhood to maturity. *J Consult Psychol* 1966;30:225–9.
45 Charlton A, Blair V. Predicting the onset of smoking in boys and girls. *Social Sci Med* 1989;29:813–18.
46 Charlton A. Anti-smoking and young people. *Modus* 1989;7:175–7.
47 Parents Against Tobacco. Fifty per cent of shops break the law by selling to under sixteens. *Parents Against Tobacco Newsletter* 1990:1:10.
48 Wilson D. *Building a tobacco blockade.* London: Health Education Authority, 1992.
49 Townsend J. Economic and health consequences of reduced smoking. In: Williams A, ed. *Health and economics.* London: Macmillan, 1987.
50 World Health Organisation. *Tobacco price and the smoking epidemic, smoke free Europe: 9.* Copenhagen: WHO, 1988.
51 Lewit EM, Coate D, Grossman M. The effects of government regulations on teenage smoking. *J Law Econ* 1981;14:545–69.
52 Townsend J. Cigarette tax, economic welfare and social class patterns of smoking. *Applied Economics* 1987;19:335–65.
53 World Health Organisation. Cigarette smuggling in Canada: an update. *Tobacco Alert* January 1993:5.
54 COMATAS. *Third report of the committee for monitoring agreements on tobacco advertising and sponsorship.* London: HMSO, 1990.
55 Aitken PP, Leathar DS, O'Hagan FJ. Children's perceptions of advertisements for cigarettes. *Social Sci Med* 1985;21:785–97.
56 Charlton A. Where there's smoke: children, televised sport and the tobacco industry. *Times Educational Supplement* 29 April 1988;3748:152.
57 Ledwith F. Does tobacco sports sponsorship on television act as advertising to children. *Health Ed J* 1984;43:85–8.
58 Piepe A, Charlton P, Morey J, White C, Yerrell P. Smoke Opera? *Health Ed J* 1986;45:199–203.
59 Taylor P. *The smoke ring: the politics of tobacco.* London: The Bodley Head, 1984:27.
60 *Confectionery and Tobacco News.* 6 November 1981.
61 Fishbein M, Ajzen J. *Belief, attitude, intention and behaviour.* New York: Addison-Wesley, 1985.
62 Becker MH, ed. *The health belief model and personal health behaviour.* New Jersey: Charles B Slack.
63 Tones BK, Tilford S, Robinson Y. *Health Education: Effectiveness and efficiency.* London: Chapman and Hall, 1990.
64 Best JA, Thompson SJ, Santi SM, Smith EA, Brown S. Preventing cigarette smoking among school children. *American Review of Public Health* 1988;9:161–201.

65 Glynn T. Essential elements of school-based smoking prevention programmes. *Journal of School Health* 1989;**59**:181–8.
66 Nutbeam D, Macaskill P, Smith C, Simpson JM, Catford J. Evaluation of two school smoking education programmes under normal classroom conditions. *BMJ* 1993;**306**:102–7.
67 Webster P, Laurance B. Cancer fear halts world sales of Perrier. *The Guardian*, 15 February, 1990.
68 Hoffmann D, Hecht SS. Advances in tobacco carcinogenesis. In: Grover P, ed. *Handbook of experimental pharmacology*. Berlin: Springer-Verlag, 1989.
69 Secretary of State for Health of Her Majesty's Government. *The health of the nation*. London: HMSO, 1992.

2 Genetic changes in lung cancer

ANTHONY BENCH, PAMELA RABBITTS

Cancer is often described as a "genetic disorder"—that is, changes within the DNA of the cells, which form the tumour—are directly responsible for the phenotypic manifestations of malignancy. Most genetic changes arise in the development of the tumour and are therefore somatic, but some are inherited and are carried in all cells of the body. Inherited genetic changes are not in themselves sufficient for the development of cancer, and so the genes involved are described as predisposing to cancer.

The complex nature of the karyotypes of lung tumour cells implies that lung cancers involve many somatic genetic changes. Some changes appear consistently and these have been well characterised. Other common solid tumours, such as breast, colon, kidney and ovary seem to involve a familiar inherited component in a subset of patients, but no such subset has been identified in patients with lung cancer. There is some evidence, however, that inherited genetic changes do have a role in the development of lung cancer.

Genetic predisposition to lung cancer

Despite the close association between smoking and lung cancer only 15% of male smokers will contract the disease.[1] The remaining 85% may have an inherited resistance to the disease. Conversely, the small number of non-smokers who develop lung cancer may be inherently susceptible. An inherited basis is difficult to prove, however, because of the overriding effects of environmental factors. The putative predisposing gene is also unlikely to be fully

19

penetrant. For example, even if a gene increases the risk of cancer 100 times (from 1 in 1000 to 1 in 10), a gene frequency of 0·1 results in a relative risk of only 2–3.[2] Large numbers of cases are required to show significance.

Epidemiological studies

Studies comparing the likelihood of lung cancer for relatives of patients with lung cancer with that for relatives of controls have shown an increased risk for relatives of patients.[3] Ooi *et al*[4] observed a 2·4 fold risk for first degree relatives of patients with lung cancer, after taking into account the effects of age, sex, pack-years, and occupational exposure. In some cases the risk was greater for non-smoking relatives of patients,[3] suggesting an inherited component. This conclusion must be treated with caution, however, as it is difficult to match controls for similar environmental exposure. Relatives of patients with the disease are also more likely to smoke[3] and are more likely to be subjected to the effects of passive smoking. In other words relatives share a similar environment, as well as genetic make-up, with patients with lung cancer.

One study has shown that the inheritance of a major gene with two codominant alleles affecting the age of onset of lung cancer fitted the pattern of disease of the 337 families in the study.[5] It was further postulated, on the basis of tobacco consumption before and after World War I, that most lung cancers in this study occurred among such gene carriers.[6]

Familial clustering

Given the high incidence of lung cancer, chance alone could account for the few instances of lung cancer families. Alveolar cell carcinoma, which is less closely linked to smoking, has been observed in one set of twins[7]; squamous cell in four out of eight siblings.[8] Different histological subtypes were observed in four of eight siblings.[9] Lung cancer has been observed in five out of 10 siblings who were part of a cancer prone family.[10] The value of such families in assessing the contribution of inherited predisposition in the development of lung cancer is limited because all those siblings who contracted lung cancer smoked, and in some cases smoked heavily.

Lung cancer has been observed in some families with the Li-Fraumeni syndrome.[11] This is a cancer prone condition due to a germline mutation of the p53 gene (TP53) on chromosome 17p13. TP53 is somatically mutated in both small cell and non-small cell carcinomas.[12] Relatives of patients with retinoblastoma, who are known to be carriers of the mutated retinoblastoma gene are at a 15-fold increased risk of developing lung cancer.[13] The retinoblastoma gene is inactivated in some small cell carcinomas.[14] An inherited mutation in the TP53 or retinoblastoma genes may predispose to lung cancer.

Ecogenetics and lung cancer

Individuals may be predisposed to a particular cancer due to increased susceptibility to the effects of certain carcinogens. In several cases an association has been found between an increased risk of cancer and a particular phenotype. For example, slow acetylators have an increased risk of bladder cancer due to arylamines.[15] This is an example of ecogenetics—the interaction of environmental insults with inherited genetic susceptibility.[16]

Most carcinogens are activated to an intermediate moiety before being broken down and excreted (figure 1).[1] Increased activity of phase I enzymes and decreased activity of phase II enzymes may predispose an individual to the effects of the carcinogen, such as the formation of carcinogen–DNA adducts, leading to DNA mutation. Inability to repair damaged DNA may also result in an increased risk of uncontrolled growth. An association between extensive metabolisers of debrisoquine and an increased risk of lung cancer has been reported.[17-20] The gene responsible has been

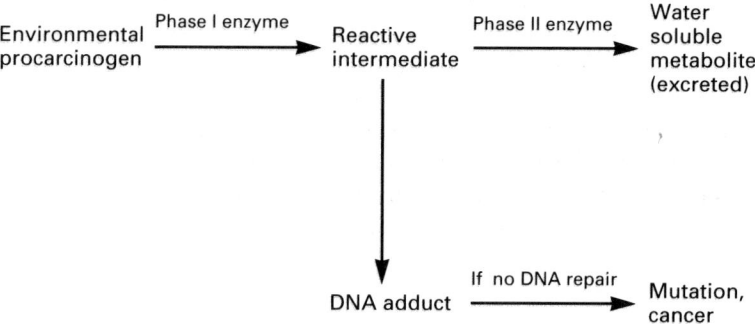

Figure 1   Simplified diagram to show route of carcinogen metabolism leading to DNA mutation.[1]

21

cloned,[21] but the observed polymorphisms have not totally correlated with the phenotype.[22] The locus (CYP2D6) probably affects the metabolism of a component of tobacco smoke to a carcinogenic form, or is in linkage disequilibrium with the true susceptibility gene.[23]

Patients with lung cancer who were presumed to be predisposed (early age of onset, non-smokers, or with an affected first degree relative) showed enhanced formation of benzo(a)pyrene–DNA adducts.[24] There is some evidence for an inherited basis to the variation in this adduct formation.[25] Similarly, the gene encoding an isozyme of glutathione transferase, a phase II enzyme, is inherited in a Mendelian manner. Lack of this isozyme is associated with increased risk of lung cancer.[26]

Differences in the ability to repair damaged DNA may also influence genetic susceptibility. There is some evidence for differences among individuals, which may be inherited, in the activities of the repair enzymes uracil DNA glycosylase, O^6-methylguanine-DNA methyltransferase, and O^6-alkylguanine-DNA-alkyltransferase.[27 28]

Genetic linkage studies

Pointers to a genetic predisposition include one or more first degree relatives with lung cancer, an early age of onset, and multiple primary neoplasms.[2 29 30] Linkage studies of the small number of families may pinpoint a predisposition locus. Because of the relatively high incidence of the disease, families with three or more lung cancer sufferers who do not smoke, or who are not subjected long term to other environmental insults, will provide more compelling evidence for a true inherited component. So far, no families of this kind have been identified. A large number of kindreds with many members showing ovarian and breast cancers,[31 32] neurofibromatosis,[33 34] or malignant melanoma[35] have been crucial in the identification of the region of the genome containing a susceptibility locus[32 35–37] and subsequent cloning of a tumour suppressor gene in the case of NF1.[38] Similar approaches for lung cancer are confounded by the high environmental input, but are not impossible.

The use of mouse genetics[39 40] and the continually improving comparative maps of man and mouse[41 42] may act as a short cut to the identification of human susceptibility genes. There is genetic evidence for the presence of three major susceptibility genes in mice.[43] One gene, Pas-1, has been mapped to distal chromosome 6,[44] a region which shows homology with human chromosomes 3p25 and 12p12–13. At the molecular level, induced mouse lung tumours resemble most closely human adenocarcinomas.[44]

Somatic genetic changes in lung cancer

Somatic genetic changes are detected in tumours by direct observation of the genetic material. Originally, this was achieved by cytogenetic analysis of chromosome spreads, obtained either from direct preparations of chromosomes from lung tumour biopsy specimens or after short term culture. The most successful studies, however, used cell lines established in culture as a source of chromosomes. Conditions for growth in vitro were established for small cell lung cancer before non-small cell lung cancer and most of the early work concentrated on this subtype. Lung tumours are often aneuploid with complex karyotypes involving several consistently observed but unidentified chromosomes. Despite this complexity deletions to the short arm of chromosome 3 were detected as a very common aberration, particularly in small cell lung cancer.

Although cytogenetic analysis allows a view of the whole genome, it is technically demanding and has largely been superseded by molecular studies.[45 46] This latter approach exploits the polymorphic variants in DNA which occur between chromosomal homologues. There are various ways in which polymorphism is generated: early studies relied on a single base change which occurred at a site recognised by a restriction enzyme. These restriction fragment length polymorphisms (RFLPs) usually only involve two allelic varients. None the less many of the early studies of lung tumour genotypes, which identified regions of allele loss, used this type of polymorphism. For later studies, which sought to define the minimal region of allele loss, a higher marker density and markers of greater informativity were required.[47] These criteria were fulfilled using the polymorphisms generated by variation between chromosomal homologues in the numbers of units in small tandem arrays of simple repeat sequences. These arrays are flanked by unique sequences for which oligonucleotide primers can be constructed to allow amplification of DNA between the priming sites to reveal any difference in the number of repeat units in the two homologous chromosomes.

23

The use of polymerase chain reaction (PCR) to analyse tumour genotypes means that very small amounts of DNA, even partially degraded, can be analysed successfully.[48] Therefore biopsy tissue stored as paraffin wax embedded blocks and sectioned on to glass slides can supply enough DNA for analysis. Using microdissection it is often possible to obtain normal and tumour cells from the same tissue section. The use of this archival material potentially allows large numbers of samples to be studied with the advantage that for many of them patient outcome is known. Rare samples are also more easily accumulated. Recently we studied somatic genetic changes in bronchial dysplastic tissue from patients with lung tumours and using archival material were also able to obtain samples of severe bronchial dysplasia from patients without invasive tumours.[49] Such samples are extremely difficult to obtain prospectively.

Specific somatic genetic changes in tumours: deletion and allele loss

The first highly consistent somatic genetic change emerged from a study of lung cancer cell lines by Whang-Peng *et al*, who observed deletions to the short arm of chromosome 3 in all the samples examined.[50] Other cytogenetic studies did not always agree with Whang-Peng's findings.[51] They were fully corroborated five years later, however, when samples of small cell lung cancer were studied by RFLP analysis and showed virtually 100% loss of alleles on 3p.[45 46] This approach was also applied to non-small cell lung cancers and, although reports vary, probably more than half of these show genetic damage to chromosome 3, with squamous cell carcinoma having the highest proportion, perhaps approaching 100%.[52 53] These studies indicate that a gene located on chromosome 3 is very important in the development of lung cancer, but it has proved difficult to locate and isolate the gene. The problem has been that, in general, deletions of 3p are very large and often the whole chromosome is lost. None the less, by using many probes which recognise polymorphisms along the length of the chromosome, three distinct, non-overlapping regions have been identified as the likely location of tumour suppressor genes involved in the development of lung cancer.[54 55] The most distal of these (3p 25) includes the location of the von Hippel-Lindau locus.[55] A recently isolated gene at this locus codes for a cancer prone syndrome, although lung cancer is not seen in the spectrum of cancers that are characteristic of afflicted families. The most proximally affected region, 3p 14→cen, is also involved in a number of other tumours, besides lung, notably breast, cervix and kidney.[56–58] A 2 Mb sequence from 3p21.3 (the third region of consistent allele loss) has been shown to be responsible for suppressing tumorigeneticity in a mouse cell line which normally forms tumours.[59] This region is therefore likely to encode a tumour suppressor gene. In independent work probes from around 3p21.3 have detected a homozygous deletion spanning less than 1 Mb in several lung tumour cell lines.[60] Homozygous deletion have been vital in both the isolation and validation of other tumour suppressor genes,[61 62] and it is likely that a candidate tumour suppressor gene will be isolated from this region in the near future.

Mutations in p53 are common in a very wide variety of tumours, including all types of lung cancer, although detected more frequently in small cell lung cancer than non-small cell lung cancer.[13] Mutations in one chromosome are usually accompanied by allele loss in the other homologue. Interestingly, the most common type of mutation of the p53 gene seen in lung cancer consists of G-T transversions.[63] Guanine residues are the preferred target for several of the mutagens found in cigarette smoke, suggesting that the p53 gene may be involved in primary carcinogenesis.[64] The biochemistry of normal and mutant p53 are being intensively studied to discover the role of the normal protein and why mutations are tumorigenic. One hypothesis is that, normally, p53 is produced at very low concentrations but damage to DNA acts as a signal to increase the concentration of p53, which prevents the cell from progressing though the cell cycle and presumably allows time for DNA repair or cell death. If p53 is altered by mutation there is no cell cycle arrest and the damaged DNA is replicated, perpetuating genetic damage which may be tumorigenic.[65]

As far as lung tumours are concerned, most attention is presently focused on 3p and the p53 genes. Other regions of the genome, however, also show consistent somatic genetic changes. Of these, damage to the retinoblastoma gene[14] is detected mainly in small cell lung cancer and, in contrast, allelic loss on 11p occurs mainly in non-small cell lung cancer.[66]

In early cytogenetic studies the same apparent chromosomal abnormality has been shown to be involved in different types of tumours, suggesting common genetic lesions even in distinct tumour types. Because genes involved in tumorigenesis have been isolated, it has been possible to test this directly. For example, abnormal retinoblastoma genes are detected in small cell lung cancer, breast cancer, osteosarcomas, soft tissue sarcomas and bladder cancer, as well as retinoblastoma.[67] Similarly, although genes confirmed as tumour suppressor genes have not been isolated from 3p, the wide range of tumours besides lung which involve 3p (breast, kidney, cervix and many more) suggests that genes on this chromosome are involved in the development of many common solid tumours.

Specific somatic genetic changes in tumours: mutations and amplification

Activation of several dominant oncogenes, often by overexpression, has been detected in lung cancer.[68] Overexpression usually occurs due to gene amplification and manifests itself visibly by the formation of unusual chromosomal structures, such as double minutes and homogeneously stained regions. Members of the *myc* gene family are often activated in lung tumours, particularly small cell lung cancer, and indeed the L-*myc* gene was first discovered in lung cancer.[69] The incidence of *myc* family involvement in lung tumours seemed to be high when cell lines were studied, but the analysis of biopsy material showed that *myc* gene amplification occurred in only about 10% of samples.[70] The normal function of these genes has remained elusive, making it difficult to suggest a mechanism whereby overexpression contributes to tumorigeneticity. Correlations of *myc* gene overexpression and prognosis have not proved informative.

By contrast, however, activation of the K-*ras* gene, which takes place by point mutation and not overexpression, does seem to be of prognostic value. These mutations are usually detected in adenocarcinoma of the lung and only in about 30% of this subtype, but patients carrying these mutations have a more aggressive clinical course.[71]

Future prospects

Considerable impediments to identifying genes which predispose to lung cancer using classic genetic approaches involving family studies remain. A more successful route might require the identification of candidate genes, such as those involved in carcinogen metabolism. Mouse strains exist which exhibit strong susceptibility to the development of lung cancer and recently this phenotype has been linked to chromosome 6 (of mice). If the gene responsible is isolated it will be useful to isolate the human homologue and to study its potential contribution to lung cancer susceptbility in man. Such a gene could be used in predictive analysis. If the gene product is involved in carcinogen metabolism the predicted risk is complicated by variability in exposure to carcinogens.

The molecular genetic analysis of lung tumours has identified highly consistent genetic changes in lung tumours. These changes may have value as markers, possibly for the early stages of the disease. These studies are more important, however, as a means of understanding the crucial steps in the tumorigenic process: a long term aim of cancer research is to devise treatments which depend on these vital differences between normal and cancer cells.

1 Law MR. Genetic predisposition to lung cancer. *Br J Cancer* 1990;**61**:195–206.
2 Ponder BAJ. Inherited predisposition to cancer. *Trends Genet* 1990;**6**:213–18.
3 Tokuhata GK, Lilienfeld AM. Familial aggregation of lung cancer in humans. *JNCI* 1963;**30**:289–312.
4 Ooi WL, Elston RC, Chen VW, Bailey-Wilson JE, Rothschild H. Increased familial risk of lung cancer. *JNCI* 1986;**76**:217–22.
5 Sellers TA, Bailey-Wilson JE, Elston RC, *et al*. Evidence for Mendelian inheritance in the pathogenesis of lung cancer. *JNCI* 1990;**82**:1272–9.
6 Sellers TA, Potter JD, Bailey-Wilson JE, Rich SS, Rothschild H, Elston RC. Lung cancer detection and prevention: Evidence for an interaction between smoking and genetic predisposition. *Cancer Res* 1992; **52** (Suppl): 2694s-7s.
7 Joishy SK, Cooper RA, Rowlery PT. Alveolar cell carcinoma in identical twins. *Ann Intern Med* 1977;**87**:447–50.
8 Brisman R, Baker RR, Elkins R, Hartmann WH. Carcinoma of lung in four siblings. *Cancer* 1967;**20**:2048–53.
9 Biran H, Goldstein J, Cohen Y. A cancer-prone kindred with four siblings afflicted by aggressive poorly differentiated bronchogenic carcinoma. *Lung Cancer* 1991;**7**:345–53.
10 Goffman TE, Hassinger DD, Mulvihill JJ. Familial respiratory tract cancer. *JAMA* 1982;**247**:1020–23.
11 Malkin D, Li FP, Strong LC, *et al*. Germ line p53 mutations in a familial syndrome of breast cancer, sarcomas, and other neoplasms. *Science* 1990;**250**:1233–8.
12 Takahashi T, Nau MM, Chiba I, *et al*. p53: A frequent target for genetic abnormalities in lung cancer. *Science* 1989;**246**:491–4.
13 Saunders BM, Jay M, Draper GJ, Roberts EM. Non-ocular cancer in relatives of retinoblastima patients. *Br J Cancer* 1989;**60**:358–65.
14 Harbour JW, Lai S-L, Whang-Peng J, Gazdar AF, Minna JD, Kaye FJ. Abnormalities in structure and expression of the human retinoblastoma gene in SCLC. *Science* 1988;**241**:353–7.
15 Hein DW. Genetic polymorphism and cancer susceptibility: Evidence concerning acetyltransferases and cancer of the urinary bladder. *Bioessays* 1988;**9**:200–4.
16 Mulvihill JJ. Host factors in human lung tumors: An example of ecogenetics in oncology. *JNCI* 1976;**57**:3–7.
17 Ayesh R, Idle JR, Ritchie JC, Crothers MJ, Hetzel MR. Metabolic oxidation phenotypes as markers for susceptibility to lung cancer. *Nature* 1984;**312**:169–70.
18 Caporaso N, Hayes RB, Dosemeci M, *et al*. Lung cancer risk, occupational exposure and the debrisoquine metabolic phenotype. *Cancer Res* 1989;**49**:3675–9.
19 Caporaso NE, Tucker MA, Hoover RN, *et al*. Lung cancer and the debrisoquine metabolic phenotype. *JNCI* 1990;**82**:1264–72.

20 Law MR, Hetzel MR, Idle JR. Debrisoquine metabolism and genetic predisposition to lung cancer. *Br J Cancer* 1989;**59**:686–7.
21 Gonzalez FJ, Skoda RC, Kimura S, *et al.* Characterization of the common genetic defect in humans deficient in debrisoquine metabolism. *Nature* 1988;**331**:442–6.
22 Sugimura H, Capraso NE, Shaw GL, *et al.* Human debrisoquine hydroxylase gene polymorphisms in cancer patients and controls. *Carcinogenesis* 1990;**11**:1527–30.
23 Shields PG, Harris CC. Molecular epidemiology and the genetics of environmental cancer. *JAMA* 1991;**266**:681–7.
24 Rüdiger HW, Nowak D, Hartmann K, Cerutti P. Enhanced formation of Benzo(a)pyrene: DNA adducts in monocytes of patients with a presumed predisposition to lung cancer. *Cancer Res* 1985;**45**:5890–4.
25 Nowak D, Schmidt-Preuss U, Jorres R, Liebke F, Rüdiger HW. Formation of DNA adducts and water-soluble metabolites of Benzo[a]pyrene in human monocytes is genetically controlled. *Int J Cancer* 1988;**41**:169–73.
26 Seidegård J, Pero RW, Millar DG, Beattie EJ. A gluathione transferase in human leukocytes as a marker for the susceptibility to lung cancer. *Carcinogenesis* 1986;**7**:751–3.
27 Vähäkangas K, Trivers GE, Plummer S, *et al.* O⁶-methylguanine-DNA methyltransferase and uracil DNA glycosylase in human broncho-alveolar lavage cells and peripheral blood mononuclear cells from tobacco smokers and non-smokers. *Carcinogenesis* 1991;**12**:1389–94.
28 Harris CC. Interindividual variation among humans in carcinogen metabolism, DNA adduct formation and DNA repair. *Carcinogenesis* 1989;**10**:1563–6.
29 Levine EG, King RA, Bloomfield CD. The role of heredity in cancer. *J Clin Oncol* 1989;**7**:527–40.
30 Hansen MF, Cavanee WK. Genetics of cancer predisposition. *Cancer Res* 1987;**47**:5518–27.
31 Claus EB, Risch N, Thompson WD. Genetic analysis of breast cancer in the cancer and steroid hormone study. *Am J Hum Genet* 1991;**48**:232–42.
32 Narod SA, Feunteun J, Lynch HT, *et al.* Familial breast–ovarian cancer locus on chromosome 17q12–q23. *Lancet* 1991;**338**:82–3.
33 Collins FS, Ponder BAJ, Seizinger BR, Epstein CJ. The von Recklinghausen neurofibromatosis region of chromosome 17-genetic and physical maps come into focus. *Am J Hum Genet* 1989;**44**:1–5.
34 Goldgar DE, Green P, Parry DM, Mulvihill JJ. Multipoint linkage analysis in neurofibromatosis type I: An international collaboration. *Am J Hum Genet* 1989;**44**:6–12.
35 Cannon-Albright LA, Goldgar DE, Meyer LJ, *et al.* Assignment of a locus for familial melanoma, MLM, to chromosome 9p13–p22. *Science* 1992;**258**:1148–52.
36 Hall JM, Lee MK, Newman B, *et al.* Linkage of early-onset familial breast cancer to chromosome 17q21. *Science* 1990;**250**:1684–9.
37 King M-C. Breast cancer genes: how many, where and who are they? *Nature Genet* 1992;**2**:89–90.
38 Wallace MR, Marchuk DA, Andersen LB, *et al.* Type 1 neurofibromatosis gene: Identification of a large transcript disrupted in three NF1 patients. *Science* 1990;**249**:181–6.
39 Chapman VM, Nadeau JH. The mouse genome: an overview. *Curr Op Genet Devt* 1992;**2**:406–11.
40 Copeland NG, Jenkins NA. Development and applications of a molecular genetic linkage map of the mouse genome. *Trends Genet* 1991;**7**:113–18.
41 Nadeau JH. Maps of linkage and synteny homologies between mouse and man. *Trends Genet* 1989;**5**:82–6.
42 O'Brien SJ, Womack JE, Lyons LA, Moore KJ, Jenkins NA, Copeland NG. Anchored reference loci for comparative genome mapping in mammals. *Nature Genet* 1993;**3**:103–12.
43 Malkinson AM, Nesbitt MN, Skamene E. Susceptibility to urethan-induced pulmonary adenomas between A/J and C57BL/6J mice: Use of AXB and BXA recombinant inbred lines indicating a three-locus genetic model. *JNCI* 1985;**75**:971–4.
44 Gariboldi M, Manenti G, Canzian F, *et al.* A major susceptibility locus to murine lung carcinogenesis maps on chromosome 6. *Nature Genet* 1993;**3**:132–6.
45 Kok KJ, Osinga B, Carritt MB, *et al.* Deletion of a DNA sequence at the chromosomal region 3p21 in all major types of lung cancer. *Nature* 1987;**330**:578–81.
46 Johnson BJ, Whang-Peng S, Naylor B, *et al.* Retention of chromosome 3 in extrapulmonary small cell cancer shown by molecular and cytogenetic studies. *JNCI* 1989;**81**:1223–8.
47 Jones M, Kazuhiro Y, Nakakmura Y. Isolation and characterisation of 19 dinucleotide repeat polymorphisms on chromosome 3p. *Hum Mol Gen* 1992;**1**:131–3.

48 Sundaresan V, Ganly P, Hasleton P, Bleehen NM, Rabbitts P. Paraffin wax-embedded material as a source of DNA for the detection of somatic genetic changes. *J Pathol* 1993;**169**:43–52.

49 Sundaresan V, Ganly P, Hasleton P, *et al*. p53 and chromosome 3 abnormalities, characteristic of malignant lung tumours, are detectable in preinvasive lesions of the bronchus. *Oncogene* 1992;**78**:1989–97.

50 Whang-Peng J, Bunn Jnr PA, Kao-Shan CS, *et al*. A non-random chromosomal abnormality, del 3p (14–23) in human small cell lung cancer (SCLC). *Cancer Genet Cytogenet* 1982;**6**:119–34.

51 Wurster-Hill DH, Cannizzaro LA, Pettengil OS, Sorenson GD, Cate, CC, Maurer LH. Cytogenetics of small cell carcinoma of the lung. *Cancer Genet Cytogenet* 1984;**13**:303–30.

52 Rabbitts P, Douglas J, Daly M, *et al*. Frequency and extent of allelic loss in the short arm of chromosome 3 in non-small cell lung cancer. *Genes Chrom Cancer* 1989;**1**:95–105.

53 Hibi K, Takahashi T, Yamakawa K, *et al*. Three distinct regions involved in 3p deletion in human lung cancer. *Oncogene* 1992;**7**:445–9.

54 Yokoyama S, Yamakawa K, Tsuchiya E, Murata M, Sakiyama S, Nakamura Y. Deletion mapping on the short arm of chromosome 3 in squamous cell carcinoma and adenocarcinoma of the lung. *Cancer Res* 1992;**52**:873–7.

55 Seizinger BR, Rouleau GA, Ozlius LJ, *et al*. Von Hippel-Lindau disease maps to the region of chromosome 3 associated with renal cell carcinoma. *Nature* 1988;**332**:268–9.

56 Sato T, Akiyama F, Sakamoto G, Kasumi F, Nakamura Y. Accumulation of genetic alterations and progression of primary breast cancer. *Cancer Res* 1991;**51**:5794–9.

57 Yokota J, Tsukada V, Nakajima T, *et al*. Loss of heterozygosity on the short arm of chromosome 3 in carcinoma of the uterine cervix. *Cancer Res* 1989;**49**:3598–601.

58 Kovacs G, Firsch S. Clonal chromosome abnormalities in tumour cells from patients with sporadic renal cell carcinomas. *Cancer Res* 1989;**49**:651–9.

59 Killary A, Wolf M, Giambernardi T, Naylor S. Definition of a tumour suppressor locus within human chromosome 3p21–22. *Proc Natl Acad Sci USA* 1992;**89**:10877–81.

60 Yamakawa K, Takahashi T, Horio Y, *et al*. Frequent homozygous deletions in lung cancer cell lines detected by a DNA marker located at 3p21.3–p22. *Oncogene* 1993;**8**:327–30.

61 Gessler M, Poutska A, Cavenee W, Neve RL, Orkin SH, Bruns GAP. Homozygous deletion in Wilms' tumours of a zinc-finger gene identified by chromosome jumping. *Nature* 1990;**343**:774–8.

62 Fearon ER, Cho KR, Nigro JM, *et al*. Identification of a chromosome 18q gene that is altered in colorectal cancers. *Science* 1990;**247**:49–56.

63 Takahashi T, Takahashi T, Suzuki H, *et al*. The p53 gene is very frequently mutated in small-cell lung cancer with a distinct nucleotide substitution pattern. *Oncogene* 1991;**6**:1775–8.

64 Mazur M, Glickman B. Sequence specificity of mutations induced by Benzo{a} Pyrene-7-8-diol-9-10-expoxide at endogenous aprt gene in CHO cells. *Som Cell Mol Gen* 1988;**14**:394–400.

65 Lane DR. p53, guardian of the genome. *Nature* 1992;**358**:15–16.

66 Shiraishi M, Morinaga S, Noguchi M, Shimosato Y, Sekiya T. Loss of genes on the short arm of chromosome 11 in human lung carcinomas. *Jpn J Cancer Res* 1987;**78**:1302–8.

67 Nordenskjöld M, Janson M, Kand M, Larsson C. Recessive mutations in the oncogenesis of retinoblastoma and multiple endocrine neoplasia type I. In: Crossman J, ed. *Molecular genetics in cancer diagnosis*. Elsevier, 1990:369–78.

68 Kaye F, Banksdale S, Harbour W, Minna J. Oncogenes in human lung cancer. In: Sluyer M, ed. *Molecular biology of cancer genes*. Ellis Horwood, 1990:207–22.

69 Nau M, Brooks B, Battey J, *et al*. L-myc a new myc-related gene amplified and expressed in human small cell lung cancer. *Nature* 1985;**318**:69–73.

70 Wong A, Ruppert J, Eggleston J, Hamilton S, Baylin S, Vogelstein B. Gene amplification of C-myc in small cell carcinoma of the lung. *Science* 1986;**233**:461–5.

71 Slebos RJC, Kibbelaar RE, Dalesio O, *et al*. K-ras oncogene activation as a prognostic marker in adenocarcinoma of the lung. *N Engl J Med* 1990;**323**:561–5.

3 Neuroendocrine differentiation in lung tumours

MARY N SHEPPARD

Many advances in what is known about neuroendocrine lung tumours have occurred over the past 20 years as a result of the application of new techniques, including electron microscopy, cell culture, immunocytochemistry, radioimmunoassay, and more recently molecular biology. These techniques have added greatly to our understanding of these complicated and often fatal tumours but they also raise many further questions, to which we do not yet have answers. For pathologists this is reflected in the multiple and at times complicated classifications applied to these tumours, depending on the techniques used and the tissues studied. For clinicians this explosion in knowledge has provided many new avenues for investigation and the possibility of developing new therapeutic tools. The subject of neuroendocrine differentiation in lung tumours is only now being unravelled. These new findings may unlock some of the secrets of lung carcinogenesis and help patients by providing diagnostic, prognostic, and possibly therapeutic information.

Neuroendocrine cells in the lung

It was Feyrter[1] in 1938 who first described clear cells in the respiratory epithelium of the human airway and included them in a "diffuse endocrine system" with other clear cells in the gastrointestinal tract and pancreas. Fröhlich[2] found that these cells were argyrophilic (taking up silver salts) and with foresight (but no evidence) he considered them to be chemoreceptors capable of monitoring gas tensions in the airways and releasing hormones. Hamperl[3] saw the similarity of these cells to the Kulschitsky or K cell of the gastrointestinal tract and suggested this name for them. Electron microscopy showed that the cells contained cytoplasmic dense core granules similar to granules found in endocrine cells elsewhere and in neurones.[4] The cells were therefore called neuro-endocrine cells to emphasise the association between the endocrine and the nervous system. Immunocytochemical and sensitive radio-immunoassay techniques confirmed the presence of several amines and peptides within these neuroendocrine cells, including sero-tonin, gastrin releasing peptide (GRP), the C flanking peptide of preproGRP, calcitonin, leu-enkephalin, calcitonin gene related peptide (CGRP), and endothelin.[5 6] Many of these peptides are also found in neurones and nerves of the central and peripheral nervous system, again showing the close link between the endocrine and nervous systems.

This widespread collection of peptide containing cells and nerves is known as the diffuse neuroendocrine system.[5 7] All these peptides have potent actions on airway smooth muscle, vasomotor tone, and airway secretion and have been proposed as important modulators of physiological changes in the lung.[8] The peptides may carry out their effects in a classic endocrine manner via the bloodstream, via nerve transmission (neuroendocrine), or in a local ("paracrine") manner. Not surprisingly, given the extensive nature of this peptide containing system in the human respiratory tract, lung tumours can produce many of these neuroendocrine features.

Neuroendocrine lung tumour classification

The secretion of what were originally considered to be "ectopic" hormones by lung tumours has been known for some time.[9] Adrenocortical overactivity leading to Cushing's syndrome was described in a patient with lung carcinoma in 1928. Sensitive assay and cell culture techniques have permitted the detection of peptide hormone secretion by tumours, particularly lung tumours,[10 11] in the absence of clinically overt syndromes. Overt endocrinological disturbance and biologically active peptide hormone production is

31

common in small cell carcinomas and carcinoid tumours; but almost all lung cancers, irrespective of histological type, are capable of producing small amounts of peptide.[12]

Both carcinoid tumours and small cell carcinomas can be recognised by light microscopy. Dense core neurosecretory granules in small cell carcinomas and carcinoid tumours added an ultrastructural feature to establish neuroendocrine differentiation[4 13] and showed the close association between these tumours and normal pulmonary endocrine cells, which also contain dense core granules. Thus both carcinoid tumours and small cell carcinomas are considered neuroendocrine tumours of the lung and included in the World Health Organisation histological classification of lung tumours.[14] This classification is based on morphological characteristics alone. Carcinoid tumours form the benign end of the spectrum and small cell carcinomas the highly malignant end. The picture becomes more complicated with the inclusion of other subgroups: several different and overlapping classifications have been introduced as a result (table I). A distinct subgroup of carcinoid tumours, labelled atypical carcinoids, with histological and clinical evidence of malignancy and with a high rate of metastases,[15] were described in 1972. These tumours form a link between carcinoid tumours and small cell carcinomas. To reflect the overlap between these tumours it was suggested that they should be reclassified as Kulschitsky cell carcinomas to indicate their spectrum of aggressiveness and emphasise their origin from the pulmonary endocrine or Kulschitsky cell[16] (table I).

Immunocytochemical techniques using antibodies to general neuroendocrine markers, including neurone specific enolase,[17] PGP 9·5, synaptophysin, and chromogranin,[18 19] were applied to neuroendocrine lung tumours by ourselves and others. Sensitive radioimmunoassay techniques were also used to detect these markers in serum and monitor tumour progression and recurrence.[20 21] More recently the application of antibodies to the neural cell adhesion molecule, NCAM, have proved useful, but this application is limited to frozen tissue.[22]

These new techniques clarified the neuroendocrine nature of the tumours, suspected from light microscopy, and produced some unexpected findings, which at first were difficult to explain. The presence of dense core granules, peptide or amine hormone production, and neuroendocrine immunocytochemical markers in undifferentiated large cell carcinomas, squamous cell carcinomas,

TABLE I Classification of pulmonary endocrine neoplasms

WHO classification[14]	WHO with IASLC modifications (Hirsch)[57]	Paladugu[16]	Gould[27]	Mosca[29]
Carcinoid tumour Atypical carcinoid tumour	Carcinoid tumour Atypical carcinoid tumour	KCC I KCC II	Carcinoid tumour Well differentiated neuroendocrine carcinoma	NEC of carcinoid type Well differentiated neuroendocrine carcinoma
Oat cell type of small cell carcinoma	small cell carcinoma	Small cell type of KCC III	Neuroendocrine carcinoma of small cell type	Neuroendocrine carcinoma of small cell type
Intermediate type of small cell carcinoma		Intermediate type of KCC III	Neuroendocrine carcinoma of intermediate type	Neuroendocrine carcinoma of intermediate (poorly differentiated type)
	Small cell/large cell carcinoma			
Combined type of small cell carcinoma	Combined type of small cell carcinoma	Combined type of KCC III	Neuroendocrine carcinoma of combined type	Combined type of neuroendocrine carcinoma

KCC: Kulschitsky cell carcinoma; NEC: Neuroendocrine carcinoma and adenocarcinomas gave rise to the concept of atypical endocrine tumours,[23][24] non-small cell carcinomas with neuroendocrine features,[25] and large cell neuroendocrine tumours of the lung.[26] These categories have caused much confusion among pathologists and clinicians concerning their behaviour, prognosis, and response to treatment.

The important question is whether these tumours with neuroendocrine features behave aggressively like small cell carcinomas and whether they therefore respond to chemotherapy. Alternatively, is neuroendocrine differentiation of no significance, merely reflecting the general heterogeneity of lung tumours? Another possibility is that neuroendocrine differentiation may indicate a more benign behaviour as typical carcinoid tumours, which display many neuroendocrine features, are usually indolent.

In an attempt to answer these questions Gould[27] suggested a spectrum comprising several related but distinct types of neuroendocrine neoplasms in the lung (table I). These studies were based on histological, immunocytochemical, and electron microscopic investigations. The typical carcinoid tumour group was retained, but Gould was quite specific about its bland nature and lack of malignancy at light microscopy. He labelled atypical carcinoids as well differentiated neuroendocrine carcinomas to emphasise their malignant behaviour. Small cell carcinomas are categorised as neuroendocrine carcinoma of small cell type. In addition, he introduced a new category, which he called neuroendocrine carcinoma of intermediate cell type, and included many large cell undifferentiated carcinomas and tumours with squamous and glandular differentiation in this group. His clinical follow up of patients with these tumours shows a spectrum of behaviour, the intermediate cell type behaving in a manner similar to that of the small cell type and being more aggressive than other large cell carcinomas.[28] He considered that neuroendocrine differentiation in non-small cell carcinomas indicated aggressive behaviour and suggested that chemotherapy should be assessed for such tumours.

A similar classification was proposed by Mosca et al.[29] These authors considered all endocrine tumours to be carcinomas. Typical carcinoids were termed neuroendocrine carcinoma of carcinoid type while peripheral and atypical carcinoid tumours were grouped together as well differentiated neuroendocrine carcinomas. Poorly differentiated tumours were classified as small cell or intermediate cell type.

34

These classifications are useful in delineating a spectrum of endocrine lung tumours but fall short on several points. Firstly, the description of the neuroendocrine carcinoma of intermediate cell type is too vague and non-specific to allow this to be separated from other undifferentiated tumours by light microscopy in my experience. Secondly, it is unfortunate that this category was named intermediate cell type as it is often confused with the "intermediate" small cell carcinoma subgroup of the WHO classification.[14] Thirdly, the classification presupposes a histogenetic relationship that has not yet been established. There is now sufficient evidence to regard carcinoid tumours as separate from small cell carcinomas and other lung tumours. Carcinoid tumours occur in a younger population and are not related to smoking habits or other risk factors for the more common forms of lung cancer. Furthermore, small cell carcinomas are rarely seen in association with carcinoid tumours. The initial response of a small cell carcinoma to combination chemotherapy and the poor long term prognosis, contrast with the chemoresistance and good prognosis of most carcinoid tumours. The use of the term Kulschitsky, which is applied to gastrointestinal endocrine cells, is confusing when applied to the lung, where both the cells and tumours are different. These observations call into question the value of attempts to devise a terminology for a spectrum of neuroendocrine tumours and the classification of these tumours remains in a state of flux.

Difficulties in the diagnosis of neuroendocrine lung tumours

The more recent classifications of neuroendocrine lung tumours are difficult for pathologists to apply, particularly for the non-small cell types. Classification requires basic light microscopy plus electron microscopy and the use of immunocytochemical markers, which are expensive and time consuming. A patient with an unusual lung tumour suspected of being a neuroendocrine tumour should probably be referred to a specialist centre for appropriate investigations; formal follow up is essential to establish long term behaviour and prognosis of the tumour.

A second problem is that lung tumours show heterogeneity with both light microscopy and electron microscopy, which can lead to problems in interpreting neuroendocrine features. Up to 7% of lung tumours have a mixed morphology according to light microscopic appearances. Multiple sampling of a tumour by electron microscopy may reveal glandular, squamous, and neuroendocrine areas even within the same cell. The clinical importance of large or small areas of neuroendocrine differentiation in a mixed tumour remains to be assessed. For definitive diagnosis large quantities of tissue may be required for special investigations. This may be a problem with bronchial biopsy, the only diagnostic technique used for many lung tumours when they are inoperable. Most neuroendocrine classifications rely heavily on the architecture of the cells within the tumour and this may not be seen easily in small biopsy specimens. Crush artefact, cellular distortion, and degeneration may make it difficult at times to separate carcinoid tumours from small cell carcinomas, a fact of great importance for treatment and prognosis.

At electron microscopy the definition of a dense core neurosecretory granule, the hallmark of neuroendocrine differentiation, is not clear and several studies show a wide divergence in the size, shape, and distribution of these granules. Differentiating them from small lysosomes may be difficult.

Finally, the specificity of the general neuroendocrine markers has been questioned as these markers have been found in non-neuroendocrine tumours, such as breast or kidney tumours. The use of only one marker for immunocytochemical diagnosis of neuroendocrine differentiation is open to criticism and a panel of markers is now recommended.

Carcinoid tumours of the lung

About 12% of all carcinoids arise in the lung but less than 1% of lung tumours are carcinoid.[30] Hamperl[3] was the first to separate carcinoids from other bronchial adenomas and point out their similarity to gastrointestinal carcinoids. The highest incidence occurs in the 31–40 year age group, with a female preponderance (62%). The tumour usually arises in a main bronchus (85%) but may be peripheral (15%).[31] Multicentric growths scattered throughout the lung have been described[32] and carcinoids can be associated with endocrine tumours elsewhere as part of a pluriglandular syndrome.[33]

Carcinoids usually protrude into the bronchus as polypoid smooth masses and have a yellow or tan colour on sectioning.

Often the tumour has an "iceberg" appearance, with much of the tumour infiltrating beneath the surface of the bronchus into the surrounding lung: care must be taken to ensure complete resection.

Histology of carcinoids

Carcinoid tumours contain uniform cells with small round to oval nuclei, few nucleoli, and granular eosinophilic cytoplasm. The cells are most commonly in islands interweaving with one another in a mosaic pattern, as interconnecting ribbons of cells in a trabecular pattern (figure 1), or in an adenopapillary pattern; mixed forms are also seen.[34] Spindle cells[35] as well as glandular differentiation, bone, and cartilage also occur. In a typical carcinoid nuclear pleomorphism and mitoses are rare. This is controversial, however, as some authors believe that the mitotic rate is very important in differentiating typical from atypical carcinoid tumours,[36] and what is the definition of "rare"?

At the ultrastructural level the main feature of all carcinoids is the large numbers of dense core neurosecretory granules in the

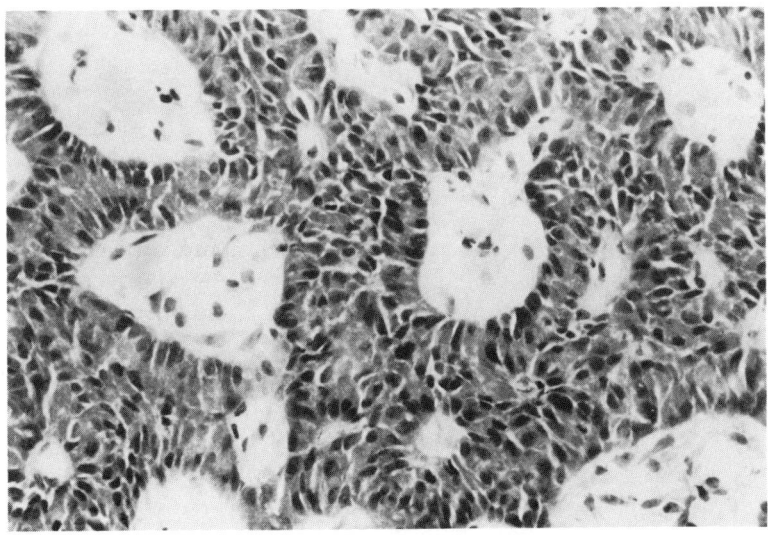

Figure 1   Typical carcinoid tumour of lung with islands and ribbons (trabeculae) of cells showing uniformity of nuclei and cytoplasm. There is hyperchromatism of the nuclei at the periphery of the islands.

cytoplasm of virtually all tumour cells[4] (figure 2). Most carcinoid tumours are strongly immunoreactive for general neuroendocrine markers (figure 3), and immunocytochemical methods and radio-immunoassay show that bronchial carcinoids produce a wide range of amines and peptide hormones.[12 27] Gould[27] found that 5-hydroxy-tryptamine was the most frequently occurring immunoreactive substance in pulmonary carcinoids, followed in descending order of frequency by gastrin releasing peptide, vasoactive intestinal polypeptide, leu-enkephalin, somatostatin, calcitonin, and adreno-corticotrophic hormone. A single tumour may produce several peptides as well as 5-hydroxytyptamine. The latter has been put forward as an immunocytochemical marker of carcinoids but is found in only half of foregut carcinoids, which limits its diagnostic usefulness.[37] S-100 positive sustentacular cells have been reported in pulmonary carcinoids[39] and labelled as "parangloid" carcinoids. The feature that distinguishes these from the rare primary pulmonary paraganglioma is that paragangliomas rarely express keratin and are strongly immunoreactive for neurofilaments.[39]

Carcinoid tumours are generally easy to diagnose by light microscopy, but the variable histological pattern can sometimes cause difficulty. It is important to diagnose them correctly as they have an excellent prognosis with a 96% five year survival if

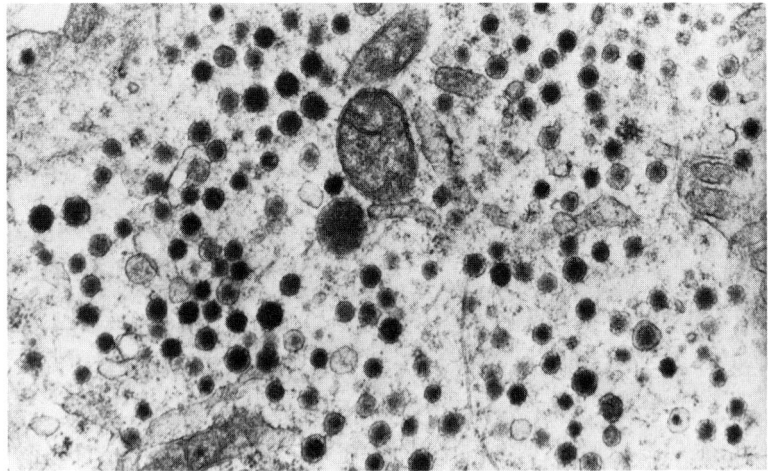

Figure 2   Dense granules in the cytoplasm of a carcinoid tumour cell. (Electron micrography by A Dewar, National Heart and Lung Institute).

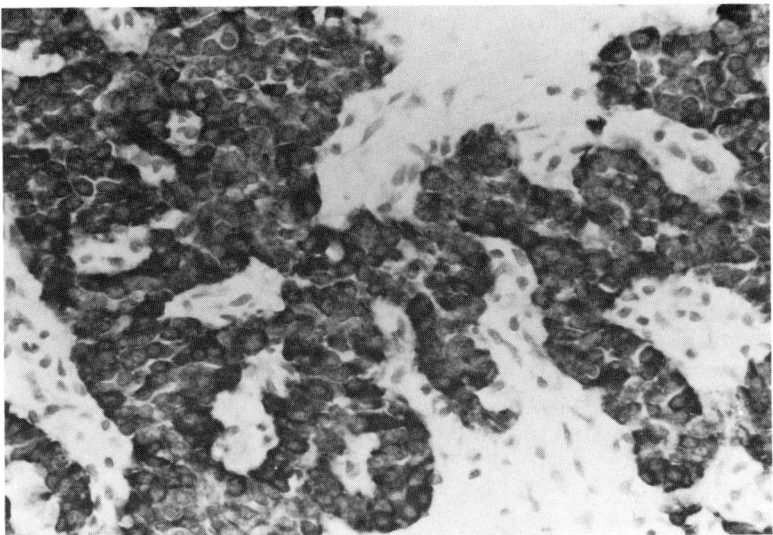

Figure 3   Positive immunostaining for chromogranin A in the cell cytoplasm of a carcinoid tumour.

confined to the lung.[30][40] Fifteen per cent of cases with no features of malignancy, however, metastasise to local lymph nodes and 5% have distant metastases.[15] Stage influences survival: 71% of patients survive after five years with lymph node metastases but only 11% with distant metastases. The behaviour of individual tumours cannot be predicted from histology alone. The early study[30] did not go into detail on the histology of the tumours, however, and studies carried out before the description of atypical carcinoid might have included these tumours. The more recent study[40] separates off atypical carcinoids and shows their worse prognosis. Even with metastases, patients can survive for long periods of time without progression of their tumour. Carcinoids are usually chemoresistant unlike small cell carcinomas. Deeply invasive tumours,[41] tumours greater than 3·0 cm in diameter, and lymph node metastases predispose to recurrence.[42]

Atypical carcinoid tumours

Arrigoni[15] first identified a group of tumours with a carcinoid architecture but with evidence of malignancy, characterised by nuclear pleomorphism, mitoses, and necrosis. He called them atypical carcinoids, but they are also known as pleomorphic or malignant carcinoids. The tumours were larger and more likely to be peripheral, and their behaviour was more aggressive than that of typical carcinoids, with regional or distant metastases in 70% of patients and a mortality of 30% after five years.

Histology

Arrigoni described atypical carcinoids as having increased pleomorphic nuclei, larger nuclei, prominent nucleoli, hyperchromatism, nuclear crowding and disorganisation with areas of tumour necrosis (figure 4). It was emphasised that these changes could be focal and that multiple sampling was needed to assess these features. He stated that an average of one to two mitoses per high power field was sufficient to label a tumour atypical, but he did not mention the actual number of mitoses in all his cases.[15]

Prognosis

Both the behaviour and prognosis of these tumours have provoked controversy. A study by Mills et al[43] showed greater mitotic

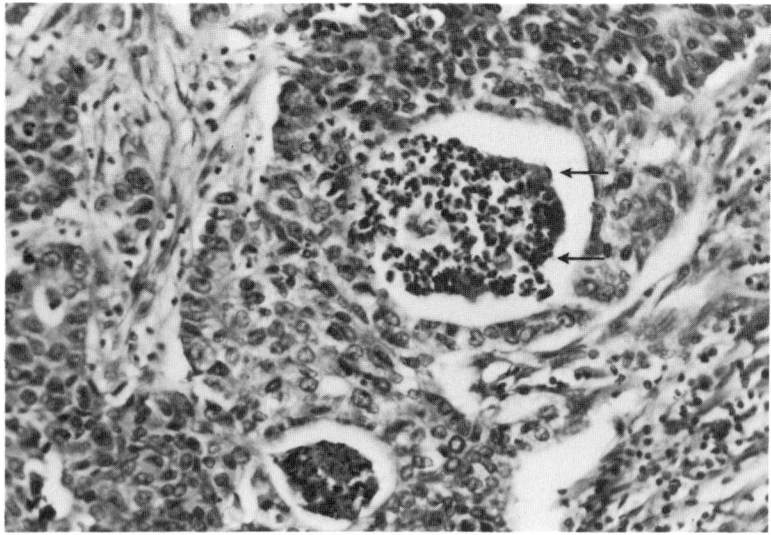

Figure 4   Atypical carcinoid tumour showing trabecular pattern and central areas of necrosis (arrows).

activity in these tumours than earlier cases, ranging from two to 28 mitoses per field. Their cases had a 50% mortality after five years but mitotic activity bore no relation to prognosis. Gould[27] was the first to label atypical carcinoids as well differentiated neuroendocrine carcinomas to emphasise their tendency towards metastases and increased mortality compared with typical carcinoids. He later subdivided them according to their degree of mitotic activity ranging from one to 40 mitoses per 10 high powered fields into three subgroups, with the implication that this had prognostic value, but the numbers were small. Follow up showed that 10 of 15 patients survived without disease while the five who developed metastases survived for long intervals, indicating a much better prognosis than that for small cell carcinoma.[44] Travis et al[36] stated that an atypical carcinoid could have up to 10 mitoses/10 high powered fields, but more than this and the tumour should be labelled a large cell neuroendocrine carcinoma. Interestingly, in two studies that examined stage 1 resectable tumours, diagnosed initially as small cell or large cell undifferentiated carcinomas, 25%[45] and 80%[46] turned out to be atypical carcinoids or well differentiated neuroendocrine carcinomas. These tumours were associated with a very much better survival at two years (60–75%) than small cell carcinomas even when these were resectable (9%). The improved survival described for stage 1 resectable small cell carcinoma[47 48] and the subsequent resurgence of interest in resecting small cell carcinomas must be looked at closely in view of these findings. Strict criteria must be used when labelling any peripheral lung lesion as a small cell carcinoma. In a more recent study[40] the mortality for atypical carcinoid was high: 60% of patients died of tumour within five years. The prognosis for these tumours, therefore, while better than that for small cell carcinoma seems at present somewhat unpredictable. Numbers have been small and co-ordinated studies are needed to clarify further the classification and behaviour of these tumours.

Dense core neurosecretory granules are far less numerous than in true carcinoids and they tend to be smaller (80–140 nm). Intertwined cytoplasmic processes are prominent and the granules are usually concentrated there. In a typical carcinoid more than half of the cells contain granules with at least five per cell whereas atypical carcinoids possess granules in half of the cells or less with less than five per cell.[26]

These tumours are immunoreactive for many of the neuroendocrine, peptide hormone, and epithelial antigens already described for carcinoids.[9] No immunocytochemical marker, however, distinguishing this tumour from typical carcinoid or small cell carcinoma, has so far been discovered.

Small cell carcinoma

The WHO classification[14] divides small cell carcinomas into three main types:

(1) small or oat cell carcinoma, consisting of small round to elongated nuclei with finely granular chromatin, no nucleoli, and little cytoplasm (figure 5);

(2) intermediate or polygonal cell carcinoma, composed of slightly larger cells with more abundant cytoplasm and with nuclear characteristics similar to those of oat cell carcinoma;

(3) small cell combined with squamous cell carcinoma or adenocarcinoma (only about 1% of tumours fall into this category).

These tumours often produce hormonal syndromes and contain dense core neurosecretory granules at the ultrastructural level[13]

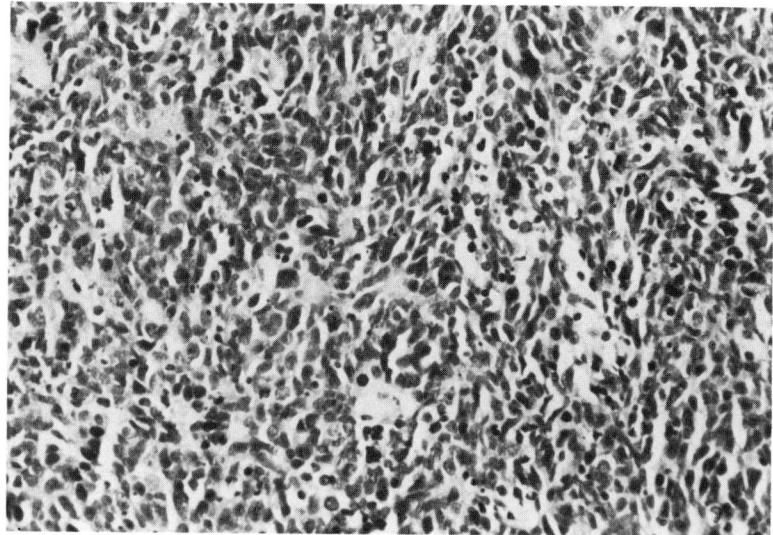

Figure 5   Small cell carcinoma of the lung showing the small hyperchromatic nuclei, nuclear moulding, little cytoplasm, and high cell death rate.

confirming their neuroendocrine nature. The granules are usually scanty and small (80–140 nm) and multiple sampling of a tumour is necessary to detect them. The use of electron microscopy has introduced new problems in the diagnosis of small cell carcinoma. Several authors report the absence of dense core granules in what appears at light microscopy to be classic small cell carcinoma. The presence of tonofilaments and desmosomes led Churg et al[49] to label them small cell squamous tumours whereas Nomori et al[50] labelled them undifferentiated carcinoma, small cell type. Patients with these tumours have been reported to survive longer than those with tumours with classic granules, but numbers of cases have been small.

There has also been controversy about the prognostic importance of the subdivisions of small cell carcinomas. Some studies have led to claims that the small cell type has a better prognosis and is more responsive to chemotherapy,[51 52] whereas others suggest that the intermediate cell type does best.[53] Two further studies suggest no difference.[54 55] This controversy, as well as the difficulty of distinguishing the small cell from the intermediate cell type histologically, has led many pathologists and clinicians to abandon this subclassification.

The mixed small cell/large cell carcinoma was first proposed as a separate entity in 1983.[56] These mixed tumours, originally thought to be rare, are being recognised more frequently especially in biopsy and necropsy specimens from patients treated intensively with radiation or chemotherapy. They represent 5–12% of all small cell carcinomas and have shown a poor response to chemotherapy with a shorter survival.[56 57]

The International Association for the Study of Lung Cancer (IASLC) has recommended that small cell carcinoma should be divided into three groups (table I):
(1) small cell carcinoma, combining the classic small cell and intermediate cell types (90% of untreated small cell carcinomas are of this type);
(2) small cell/large cell carcinoma, in which at least 24% of the cells have large granular or more open nuclei with prominent eosinophilic nucleoli (4–6% of untreated small cell carcinomas fall into this category);
(3) carcinoma of mixed type similar to WHO group 3.

This classification is supported by experimental studies on small cell carcinoma. Many continuous cell lines and xenographs have been established.[58] Most contain dense core granules, express neuroendocrine and other markers associated with small cell carcinoma, and are radiosensitive. The cytological features of these "classic" cell lines are of the small cell subtype of small cell lung carcinoma. Some small cell lines have a "variant" morphological appearance and resemble small/large cell carcinomas or large cell carcinomas. They lack dense core granules and other neuroendocrine features. They are sometimes associated with amplification of the c-*myc* oncogene and they grow more rapidly, are cloned more efficiently, and are radioresistant. These variant cell lines may develop from classic small cell carcinomas, especially if these have been treated with chemotherapy, or if they are from mixed small cell/large cell carcinomas. The development of large cell features in a small cell carcinoma after chemotherapy may be due to the treatment or to the survival of large cells already present in the tumour before treatment. There is wide support for the above classification,[59] though some studies suggest no difference in prognosis.[54]

Small cell carcinomas are immunoreactive for neuronal markers, but to a much lesser extent than the other neuroendocrine tumours. Unfortunately from the diagnostic and prognostic point of view, the more malignant the neuroendocrine tumour is, the less likely it is to give positive immunocytochemical results for neuroendocrine antigens or peptide hormones.[27]

Immunocytochemistry and radioimmunoassay provide useful data on stored and secreted peptide; information on gene expression and regulation requires molecular biology techniques, including northern and Southern blotting, in situ hybridisation, and the polymerase chain reaction. Molecular techniques have helped to elucidate some of the problems involved in the production of these peptides. Even though the protein product may not be present, such as chromogranin A, the gene is activated within the cytoplasm of tumour cells[60] (figure 6).

The peptide protein may be rapidly secreted into the circulation so that it is not detectable in the cell, or it may be rapidly degraded. Serum concentration of neuroendocrine markers, such as neurone specific enolase, have been used as tumour markers for small cell carcinoma, and they may be useful in monitoring treatment and predicting relapse.[20 21] Another immunocytochemical finding is that growth factors, such as gastrin releasing hormone, may not be expressed in small cell carcinomas, even

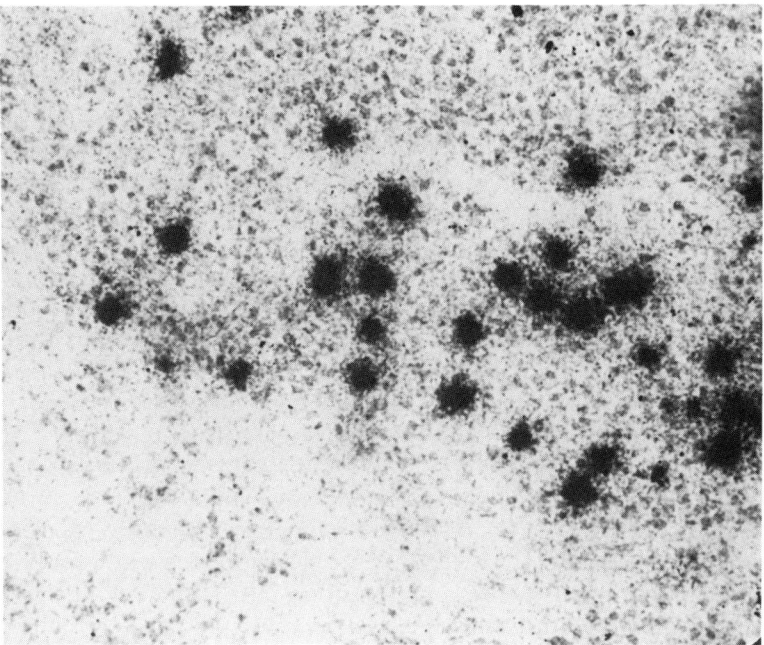

Figure 6 Small cell carcinoma of the lung giving a focal intense signal for chromogranin A messenger RNA. (From Hamid *et al*[60]; reproduced by courtesy of the *Journal of Pathology*).

though the gene is active.[61] This may be due to the production of abnormal forms of the growth factor[18] or rapid degradation.

The mechanism underlying the paraneoplastic syndromes— neuropathies, encephalomyelitis, and myopathies—is unknown, though production of antigens, similar to neuronal antigens, by the tumour and the subsequent mobilisation of antibodies by the body in response to the antigens are thought to explain many of the syndromes.[62] This suggests that many more tumour products remain to be discovered.

Non-small cell neuroendocrine carcinomas

The first description of non-small cell neuroendocrine carcinomas, which by light microscopy had been diagnosed as large cell or squamous cell carcinomas or adenocarcinomas, came in 1981,

45

when McDowell et al[23] described seven cases in the periphery of the lung. Electron microscopy subsequently showed dense core neurosecretory granules, thus establishing them as neuroendocrine tumours (in 4% of 150 lung tumours). The tumours were argyrophilic and contained 5-hydroxytryptamine, confirming endocrine differentiation at the level of light microscopy. McDowell labelled them atypical endocrine tumours of the lung. Another report[24] suggested that as many as 9% of non-small cell carcinomas in the lung contained neurosecretory granules, and that median survival and rates of response to treatment were in the ranges seen with non-small cell carcinoma. Others,[25] however, claimed that they behaved more aggressively and labelled them large cell neuroendocrine tumours or non-small cell carcinomas with neuroendocrine features. Gould[27] included them as intermediate cell type in his spectrum of neuroendocrine carcinomas and suggested that cell nesting with peripheral palisading of nuclei would help to identify this tumour by light microscopy, a point emphasised by Mooi et al.[25] Travis et al[36] emphasised that the cells are large with prominent nucleoli in the nuclei, a high mitotic rate, and a low nuclear: cytoplasmic ratio and have an organoid, trabecular, and palisading pattern, which indicate the neuroendocrine phenotype. He labelled them large cell neuroendocrine carcinomas in contrast to large cell carcinomas with neuroendocrine features—tumours in which the neuroendocrine features can be detected only by immunohistochemistry or electron microscopy. In a later study and follow up by Gould's group the tumours behaved in a manner similar to that of small cell carcinoma.[44] The clinical relevance of a separate group of non-small cell neuroendocrine carcinomas remains to be determined; most studies have been small and lacked follow up.

Specificity of neuroendocrine markers

Several workers applying neuroendocrine markers to lung tumours have found that a proportion of all tumour types give positive results.[63] This may reflect the heterogeneity of lung tumours; others consider that the markers lack specificity for neuroendocrine tumours.[64] We found that, although neurone specific enolase and PGP + 9.5 are positive in most neorendocrine tumours, they are also present in 10–30% of non-neuroendocrine lung tumours and are not now considered reliable markers of neuroendocrine differentiation. Chromogranin A, Leu-7, and synaptophysin appear to be more useful markers but they stain fewer neuroendocrine tumours than neurone specific enolase and PGP9.5. More recently NCAM has been proposed as the best immunohistochemical predictor of neuroendocrine differentiation.[65] Use of a panel of markers rather than a single marker is advised, with a combination of neurone specific enolase, PGP9.5, chromogranin, and synaptophysin and NCAM being the best. A positive result with two of the four markers is recommended before a tumour can be labelled as neuroendocrine.

Oncogenes and anti-oncogenes in neuroendocrine tumours

Oncogenes and anti-oncogenes and abnormalities in their expression have been detected in neuroendocrine tumours. The major oncogenes implicated in neuroendocrine tumours are the *myc* and *ras* families. *Myc* amplification seems to be associated with tumour progression rather than pathogenesis. C-*jun* is also amplified in small cell lung cancer.[66]

Restriction fragment length polymorphism (RFLP) analysis indicates that deletions of chromosome arms 3p, 13q, and 17p are common in small cell lung cancer. Chromosome 13q is the site of the retinoblastoma gene and the protein product of this is absent in small cell lung cancer, indicating mutation.[67] 17q is the location of the p53 gene whose protein product is abnormally expressed in small cell carcinoma[67]; 3p is the site of an as yet unidentified anti-oncogene.

Conclusion

Neuroendocrine lung tumours are proving a fruitful area of research for understanding the basic mechanisms of carcinogenesis. Rapid advances in the molecular and cell biology of these tumours should help to determine their spectrum of behaviour. New studies are essential, using light microscopy, electron microscopy, immunocytochemistry, and molecular biology techniques, for clarifying different subtypes and designing future treatments, particularly now that many growth factors are known to be produced by these tumours. A classification based on morphological and functional criteria may prove to be of therapeutic importance in the future.

1 Feyrter F. *Ueber diffuse endokrine epitheliale Organe.* Leipzig, Bath, 1938.
2 Fröhlich F. Die "Helle Zelle" der Bronchialschleim hautaud ihre Beziehungen zum problem der Chemoreceptoren. *Frankfurt Z Pathol* 1949;**60**:517–59.
3 Hamperl H, Uber G. Bronchial tumoren (cylindrome und carcinoide). *Virchows Arch (Pathol Anat)* 1937;**300**:46–8.
4 Bensch KG, Gordon GB, Miller LR. Electron microscopic and biochemical studies on the bronchial carcinoid tumour. *Cancer* 1965;**18**:592–602.
5 Springall DR, Polak JM. Localization of peptides in the lung. In: Piper PJ, ed. *Advances in the understanding and treatment of asthma.* New York: Academy of Sciences, 1991:1–20.
6 Giaid A, Polak JM, Gaitonde V, *et al.* Distribution of endothelin-like immunoreactivity and mRNA in the developing and adult human lung. *Am J Respir Cell Mol Biol* 1991;**4**:50–8.
7 Polak JM, Bloom SR. Occurrence and distribution of regulatory peptides in the respiratory tract. In: Havemann K, Sorenson G, Gropp C, eds. *Recent results in cancer research.* Berlin: Springer, 1985:1–16.
8 Becker KL. Lung cancer: Peptide hormones and their possible functions in the normal and abnormal lung. In: Kavemann K, Sorenson G, Gropp C, eds. *Recent results in cancer research.* Berlin: Springer, 1985:17–28.
9 Brown WH. A case of pluriglandular syndrome. *Lancet* 1928;**ii**:1022–3.
10 Ratcliffe JG, Podmore J. Ectopic hormones. In: Boelsma E, Rumke P, eds. *Tumour markers: impact and prospects.* Amsterdam: North Holland Biomedical Press, 1979:3–23.
11 Baylin SB, Mendelsohn G. Ectopic (inappropriate) hormone production by tumours: mechanisms involved and the biological and clinical implications. *Endocrinol Rev* 1980;**1**:45–77.
12 Kameya Y, Kodama T, Shimosato Y. Morphology of lung cancer in relation to its function. In: Shimosato Y, Melamed MR, Nettesheim P, eds. *Morphogenesis of lung cancer.* 2nd Edn. Florida: CRC Press, 1982: 107–29.
13 Bensch KG, Corrin B, Pariente R, Spencer H. Oat cell carcinoma of the lung: its origin and relationship to bronchial carcinoid. *Cancer* 1968;**22**:1163–72.
14 World Health Organization, The World Health Organization histological typing of lung tumors. Second edition. *Am J Clin Pathol* 1982;**77**:123–36.
15 Arrigoni MG, Woolner LB, Bernatz PE. Atypical carcinoid tumours of the lung. *J Thorac Cardiovasc Surg* 1972;**64**:413–21.
16 Paladugu RR, Benfield JR, Pak HY, Ross RK, Teplitz RL. Bronchopulmonary Kulchitzky cell carcinomas. A new classification scheme for typical and atypical carcinoids. *Cancer* 1985;**55**:1303–11.
17 Sheppard MN, Corrin B, Bennett MH, Marangos PJ, Bloom SR, Polak JM. Immunocytochemical localisation of neuron-specific enolase in small cell carcinoma and carcinoid tumours of the lung. *Histopathology* 1984;**8**:171–81.
18 Addis BJ, Hamid Q, Ibrahim NBN, Fahey M, Bloom SR, Polak JM. Immunohistochemical markers of small cell carcinoma and related neuroendocrine tumours of the lung. *J Pathol* 1987;**153**:137–50.
19 Wiedenmann B, Huttner WB. Synaptophysin and chromogranins/secretogranins—Widespread constituents of distinct types of neuroendocrine vesicles and new tools in tumour diagnosis. *Virchows Arch (Cell Pathol)* 1989;**58**:95–121.
20 Carney DN, Ihde DC, Cohen MH, Marangos PJ, Bunn PA, Minna JD. Serum neuron-specific enolase: a marker for disease extent and response to therapy of small-cell lung cancer. *Lancet* 1982;**ii**:583–5.
21 Burghuber OC, Worofka B, Schernthaner G, *et al.* Serum neuron-specific enolase is a useful tumour marker for small cell lung cancer. *Cancer* 1990;**65**:1386–90.
22 Broers JL, Mijnheere EP, Rot MK, *et al.* Novel antigens characteristic of neuroendocrine malignancies. *Cancer* 1991;**67**:619–33.
23 McDowell EM, Wilson TS, Trump BS. Atypical endocrine tumours of the lung. *Arch Pathol Lab Med* 1981;**105**:20–8.

24 Neal MH, Kosinski R, Cohen P, Ohrenstein JM. Atypical endocrine tumours of the lung. A clinicopathologic study of 19 cases. *Hum Pathol* 1986;**17**:1264–77.
25 Mooi WJ, Dewar A, Springall DR, Polak JM, Addis BJ. Non-small cell lung carcinomas with neuroendocrine features. A light microscopic, immunohistochemical and ultrastructural study of 11 cases. *Histopathology* 1988;**13**:329–37.
26 Hammond ME, Sause WT. Large cell neuroendocrine tumours of the lung. *Cancer* 1985;**56**:1624–9.
27 Gould VE, Linnoila RI, Memoli VA, Warren WH. Neuroendocrine cells and neuroendocrine neoplasms of the lung. In: Sommers SC, Rosen PP, eds. *Pathology Annual*. Connecticut: Century-Crofts, 1983:287–330.
28 Warren WH, Gould VE. Neuroendocrine neoplasm of the bronchopulmonary tract. *J Thorac Cardiovasc Surg* 1985;**89**:819–25.
29 Mosca L, Ceresoli A, Anzanello E, *et al*. Neuroendocrine structures in normal and diseased human lung. *Applied Pathology* 1986;**4**:147–61.
30 Godwin JD. Carcinoid tumours. *Cancer* 1975;**36**:560–9.
31 Oike N, Bernatz PE, Woolner LB. Carcinoid tumours of the lung. *Ann Thorac Surg* 1976;**22**:270–7.
32 Skinner C, Ewen SWB. Carcinoid lung: diffuse pulmonary infiltration by a multifocal bronchial carcinoid. *Thorax* 1976;**31**:212–19.
33 Williams ED, Celestin LR. The association of bronchial carcinoid and pluriglandular adenomatosis. *Thorax* 1962;**17**:120–7.
34 Jones RA, Dawson IMP. Morphology and staining patterns of endocrine tumours in the gut, pancreas and bronchus and their possible significance. *Histopathology* 1977;**1**:137–50.
35 Nelson EL, Houghton DC. Concurrent spindle cell peripheral pulmonary carcinoid tumor and Merkel cell tumor of the skin. *Arch Pathol Lab Med* 1990;**114**:420–3.
36 Travis WD, Linnoila RI, Tsokos MG. Neuroendocrine tumors of the lung with proposed criteria for large cell neuroendocrine carcinoma. *Am J Surg Pathol* 1991;**15**:529–53.
37 Shaw PA. Comparison of immunologic detection of 5-hydroxytryptamine by monoclonal antibodies with standard silver stains as an aid to diagnosing carcinoid tumours. *J Clin Pathol* 1988;**41**:265–72.
38 Barbareschi M, Frigo B, Mosca L, *et al*. Bronchial carcinoids with S-100 positive sustentacular cells. A comparative study with gastrointestinal carcinoids, pheochromocytomas and paragangliomas. *Path Res Pract* 1990;**186**:212–22.
39 Hoefler H, Denk H, Lackinger E, Helleis G, Polak JM, Heitz PU. Immunocytochemical demonstration of intermediate filament cytoskeletal proteins in human endocrine tissues and (neuro-) endocrine tumours. *Virchows Arch (Pathol Anat)* 1986;**409**:609–29.
40 Harpole DH, Feldman JM, Buchanan S, *et al*. Bronchial carcinoid tumors—a retrospective analysis of 126 patients. *Ann Thorac Surg* 1992;**54**:50–5.
41 Hajdu SI, Winawer SJ, Myers WPL. Carcinoid tumours: a study of 204 cases. *Am J Clin Pathol* 1974;**61**:521–8.
42 McCaughan BC, Martini N, Bains MS. Bronchial carcinoids. *J Thorac Cardiovasc Surg* 1985;**89**:8–17.
43 Mills SE, Cooper PH, Walker AN, Kron IL. Atypical carcinoid tumour of the lung. *Am J Surg Pathol* 1982;**6**:643–54.
44 Warren WH, Penfield FL, Gould VE. Neuroendocrine neoplasms of the lung. A clinicopathologic update. *Thorac Cardiovasc Surg* 1989;**98**:321–32.
45 Warren WH, Memoli VA, Jordan A, Gould VE. Re-evaluation of pulmonary neoplasms resected as small cell carcinomas. Significance of distinguishing between well-differentiated and small cell neuroendocrine carcinomas. *Cancer* 1990;**65**:1003–10.
46 Kron IL, Harman PK, Mills SE. A reappraisal of limited stage undifferentiated carcinoma of the lung. *J Thorac Cardiovasc Surg* 1982;**84**:734–7.
47 Karrer K, Shields TW, Denck H, Hrabar B, Vogt-Moykopf I, Salzer GM. The importance of surgical and multimodality treatment for small cell bronchial carcinoma. *J Thorac Cardiovasc Surg* 1989;**978**:168–76.
48 Prasad US, Naylor AR, Walker WS, *et al*. Long term survival after pulmonary resection for small cell carcinoma of the lung. *Thorax* 1989;**44**:784–7.
49 Churg A, Johnston WH, Stulbuarg M. Small cell squamous and mixed small cell squamous-small cell anaplastic carcinomas of the lung. *Am J Surg Pathol* 1980;**4**:255–63.
50 Nomori H, Shimosato Y, Kodama T, Morinaga S, Nakajima T, Watanabe S. Subtypes of small cell carcinomas of the lung: morphometric ultrastructural and immunohistochemical analysis. *Hum Pathol* 1986;**17**:604–13.

51 Nixon D, Murphy GF, Sewell CW, Kutner M, Lynn MJ. Relationship between survival and histological type in small cell anaplastic carcinoma of the lung. *Cancer* 1979;**44**:1045–9.

52 Davis S, Stanley KE, Yesner R, Kuang DT, Morris JF. Small cell carcinoma of the lung—survival according to histologic sub-type. *Cancer* 1981;**47**:1863–6.

53 Katlic M, Carter D. *Prognostic implications of histology, size and location of primary tumours.* New York: Raven Press, 1979:143–50.

54 Bepler G, Neumann K, Holle R, Havemann K, Kalbfleisch H. Clinical relevance of histologic subtyping in small cell lung cancer. *Cancer* 1989;**64**:74–9.

55 Radic PA, Matthews MJ, Ihde DC, *et al.* The clinical behaviour of "mixed" small cell/large cell bronchogenic carcinoma compared to "pure" small cell subtypes. *Cancer* 1982;**50**:2894–902.

56 Hirsch FR, Osterlind K, Hansen HH. The prognostic significance of histopathologic subtyping of small cell carcinoma of the lung according to the World Health Organization classification. *Cancer* 1983;**52**:2144–60.

57 Hirsch FR, Matthews MJ, Aisner S. Histopathologic classification of small cell lung cancer: changing concepts and terminology. *Cancer* 1988;**62**:973–7.

58 Carney DN, Gazdar AF, Bepler G, *et al.* Establishment and identification of small cell lung cancer cell lines having classic and variant features. *Cancer Res* 1985;**45**:2913–23.

59 Fushimi H, Kikui M, Morino H, *et al.* Detection of large cell component in small cell lung carcinoma by combined cytologic and histologic examinations and its clinical implication. *Cancer* 1992;**70**:599–605.

60 Hamid Q, Corrin B, Sheppard MN, Polak JM. Localisation of chromogranin mRNA in small cell carcinoma of the lung. *J Pathol* 1991;**163**:293–8.

61 Hamid Q, Bishop A, Springall DR. Detection of human pro-bombesin mRNA in neuroendocrine (small cell) carcinoma of the lung. *Cancer* 1989;**63**:266–71.

62 Graus F, Elkin KB, Cordon-Cardo C, Posner JB. Sensory neuropathy and small cell lung cancer. *Am J Med* 1983;**80**:45–52.

63 Sheppard MN, Morittu L, Moss F, *et al.* A study of epithelial, neuroendocrine and natural killer cell antibodies in adult lung and lung tumours. *Lung Cancer* 1988;**4**:70–2.

64 Dranoff G, Bignen DD. A word of caution in the use of neuron-specific enolase expression in tumour diagnosis. *Arch Pathol Lab Med* 1988;**108**:535–40.

65 Brambilla E, Veale D, Moro D, Morel F, Dubois F, Brambilla C. Neuroendocrine phenotype in lung cancers. Comparison of immunohistochemical with biochemical determination of enolase isoenzymes. *Am J Clin Pathol* 1992;**98**:88–97.

66 Minna JD. Autocrine growth factor production, chromosomal delections and oncogene activation in the pathogenesis of lung cancer. *Lung Cancer* 1988;**4**:6–10.

67 Barbareschi M, Girlando S, Mauri FA, *et al.* Tumour suppressor gene products, proliferation, and differentiation markers in lung neuroendocrine neoplasms. *J Pathol* 1992;**166**:343–50.

4 Growth factors and lung cancer

PENELLA J WOLL

Growth factors are a diverse group of signalling molecules taking part in the control of cell proliferation. Whether they act on postganglionic receptors (neurotransmitters), nearby cells (autocrine and paracrine hormones), or distant target organs (endocrine hormones), they require specific receptors and intracellular signal transduction pathways to stimulate cell division. Abnormal expression of growth factors, their receptors, or their signalling pathways may result in the unrestrained growth of cancer. The finding that many such changes are associated with oncogene activation has underpinned the hypothesis that cancer results from cumulative somatic mutations.

In addition to advancing our understanding of carcinogenesis, elucidation of the action of growth factors presents exciting opportunities for the development of new therapeutic strategies against cancer. This review considers the evidence for the action of growth factors in lung cancer and the implications for treatment.

Small cell lung cancer

About a quarter of lung cancers are small cell lung cancer. They are characterised by the presence of cytoplasmic secretory granules and their ability to synthesise a wide range of peptides and hormones (table I). Among these, the bombesin related peptides, including gastrin releasing peptide, first attracted interest as putative autocrine growth factors, but many others are now known to act as mitogens in experimental systems,[1] and a more complex

51

TABLE I   Factors synthesised by small cell lung cancer

Adrenocorticotrophin	Lipotropin
Atrial natriuretic peptide	Neurotensin
Bombesin/gastrin releasing peptide neuromedin B	Oestradiol
Calcitonin	Opioid peptides
Calcitonin gene related peptide	Oxytocin
Cholecystokinin	Parathyroid hormone
Chorionic gonadotrophin	Physalaemin
Endothelin	Prolactin
Follicle stimulating hormone	Serotonin
Gastrin	Somatostatin
Glucagon	Stem cell factor
Granulocyte colony stimulating factor	Substance K
Growth hormone	Substance P
Growth hormone releasing factor	Transferrin
Insulin like growth factor I	Vasoactive intestinal peptide
Insulin like growth factor binding proteins	Vasopressin

picture is emerging of growth stimulation by multiple autocrine and paracrine loops.

Bombesin/gastrin releasing peptide

Gastrin releasing peptide (27 amino acids) is the principal mammalian homologue of the amphibian peptide bombesin (14 amino acids). It is present in neurones of the gut and central nervous system. Although it is abundant in fetal lung, with maximal expression of messenger RNA (mRNA) at 16–30 weeks, reduced concentrations are found in infants with the respiratory distress syndrome and it is sparse in adult lung.[23] These observations led to the intriguing suggestion that bombesin/gastrin releasing peptide could act as a growth factor for fetal lung.

Bombesin/gastrin releasing peptide is found in specimens and cell lines of small cell lung cancer and the concentrations correlate well with those of gastrin releasing peptide mRNA.[4–6] The finding that bombesin/gastrin releasing peptide could stimulate the growth of murine Swiss 3T3 fibroblasts focused attention on neuropeptides as possible tumour growth factors.[7] The binding of iodine-125 labelled gastrin releasing peptide to small cell lung cancer cells suggested that specific receptors are present on these cells.[8] Gastrin releasing peptide has since been shown to stimulate the growth of small cell lung cancers in vitro and in vivo.[9 10] Cuttitta et al[11] used a monoclonal antibody to bombesin to inhibit the growth of two small cell lung cancer cell lines in vitro and of one as a xenograft in nude mice. There is thus persuasive evidence that bombesin/gastrin releasing peptide can act as an autocrine growth factor in at least some small cell lung cancers.

Because of the complex interactions among growth factors in tissue preparations and in vivo, the characterisation of their individual effects has been possible only in homogeneous cell lines such as Swiss 3T3 cells. These cells attain quiescence in serum depleted medium, but resume DNA synthesis after the addition of fresh serum or purified growth factors. The mode of action of bombesin/gastrin releasing peptide has been studied in detail in these cells and serves as a paradigm of growth factor action. Swiss 3T3 cells have proved to be a robust model for small cell lung cancer because they have receptors for a range of mitogenic neuropeptides,[12] including bombesin/gastrin releasing peptide, bradykinin, endothelins, vasopressin, and vasoactive intestinal peptide.

Bombesin/gastrin releasing peptide binds to a single class of high affinity receptors on the surface of Swiss 3T3 cells.[13] The receptors are glycoproteins with a relative molecular weight of 75 000–85 000, with a core of 43 000.[14–16] They are coupled to one or more guanine nucleotide binding proteins (G proteins) as judged by the modulation of ligand binding in preparations of membranes and solubilised receptors.[12] The bombesin/gastrin releasing peptide receptor has recently been cloned and sequenced.[17 18] At least two receptor subtypes for mammalian bombesin like peptides have now been distinguished.[19] They belong to the class of G protein coupled receptors with seven predicted transmembrane helices clustered to form a ligand binding pocket.[20 21] Other neuropeptide mitogens with receptors of this type are angiotensin, endothelin, serotonin, substance K, substance P, and vasopressin.[22–25] Interestingly, angiotensin and serotonin receptors can behave like oncogenes.[26 27]

Binding of bombesin/gastrin releasing peptide to its receptor in Swiss 3T3 cells triggers a cascade of signals in the membrane, cytosol, and nucleus, culminating in DNA synthesis 10–15 hours later. One of the earliest events is a rapid mobilisation of calcium (Ca^{2+}) from intacellular stores, leading to a transient increase in the cytosolic Ca^{2+} concentration followed by Ca^{2+} efflux from the cells.[28] These changes are mediated by inositol 1,4,5-trisphosphate, which with 1,2-diacylglycerol is generated by hydrolysis of phosphatidyl inositol 4,5 bisphosphate by phospholipase C in the plasma membrane. 1,2-Diacylglycerol can also be generated from other sources, such as phosphatidylcholine hydrolysis.[29] It stimulates protein kinase C, causing phosphorylation of its major substrate, the 80K protein.[30][31] Recently, bombesin has also been shown to induce a rapid and potent stimulation of tyrosine phosphorylation in Swiss 3T3 cells.[32] The target substrates of this activity are distinct from those of the polypeptide growth factor receptors which have intrinsic tyrosine kinase activity.

Other signalling pathways activated by bombesin/gastrin releasing peptide include arachidonic acid and prostaglandin E$_2$ release, cyclic AMP production, and the rapid exchange of sodium, potassium, and hydrogen ions across the cell membrane, leading to cytoplasmic alkalinisation and increased intracellular K$^+$ concentration.[33][34] In common with many other growth factors, bombesin/gastrin releasing peptide stimulates transient expression of the nuclear oncogenes c-*fos* and c-*myc*.[35] Thus bombesin/gastrin releasing peptide triggers a complex network of signals incorporating an unusual degree of redundancy, which ensures amplification of the stimulus and suggests that it has an important role. Attempts to block growth factor action through any single pathway are unlikely to be successful, so therapeutic strategies must embrace this complexity.

Bombesin/gastrin releasing peptide signals in small cell lung cancer
Preliminary studies of the actions of bombesin/gastrin releasing peptide in small cell lung cancer suggest that the signals stimulated in these cells are similar to those seen in Swiss 3T3 cells. Rapid and transient mobilisation of intracellular Ca^{2+} occurs, with inositol phosphate turnover.[36][37] We therefore tested the hypothesis that small cell lung cancer cells express receptors for numerous mitogenic neuropeptides.

We screened 32 peptides and hormones for their ability to mobilise intracellular Ca^{2+} in five small cell lung cancer cell lines.[38] The cells were incubated with the fluorescent Ca^{2+} indicator Fura-2, washed and resuspended in a cuvette in a continuously recording luminescence fluorimeter. All the cell lines responded to addition of peptide with rapid and transient mobilisation of intracellular Ca^{2+}, but the active peptides differed between the cell lines. Three cell lines responded to gastrin releasing peptide whereas all cell lines responded to vasopressin. Responses were also obtained with bradykinin, cholecystokinin, galanin, and neurotensin. The cells lost their responsiveness with repeated additions of the same peptide, but retained the ability to respond to unrelated peptides (homologous desensitisation). Their effects were blocked by ligand specific antagonists. These observations indicate that the peptides act through distinct receptors and that small cell lung cancer cells have specific receptors for many peptides.

Additional factors have now been shown to bind to small cell lung cancer cells or stimulate intracellular signals, such as calcium mobilisation and inositol phosphate turnover (table II). Many of these are neuropeptides and most can be synthesised by small cell lung cancers (table I). All are known to act as growth promoting or inhibiting factors under appropriate conditions.[1] These findings have dramatically altered our view of growth control in small cell lung cancers. Less than ten years ago bombesin/gastrin releasing peptide was hailed as an autocrine growth factor for these cells. Now we envisage a complex network of autocrine and paracrine growth factors secreted by these tumours, interacting with tumour and host cells to support proliferation. Stimulation of tumour growth by these factors was necessary to confirm this hypothesis.

TABLE II Factors that bind to small cell lung cancer cells or initiate signalling

Bombesin/gastrin releasing peptide neuromedin B
Bradykinin
Cholecystokinin
Galanin
Gastrin
Granulocyte colony stimulating factor
Granulocyte-macrophage colony stimulating factor
Insulin like growth factor I
Neurotensin
Opioid peptides
Physalaemin
Somatostatin
Stem cell factor
Tachykinins
Testosterone
Transferrin
Vasoactive intestinal peptide
Vasopressin

Growth stimulation of small cell lung cancer

The number of secreted factors, which have clearly been shown to stimulate small cell lung cancer proliferation, is increasing rapidly (table III). Bombesin like peptides, including gastrin releasing peptide and neuromedin B, stimulate the growth of small cell lung cancer colonies in soft agar in vitro[9][39] but not in liquid culture, probably because maximal growth is already achieved in serum free HITES medium.[40] In nude mice bearing human small cell lung cancer xenografts and having thrice daily intraperitoneal injections of bombesin, tumour size and weight increased more than in a control group injected with saline.[10]

Vasopressin Vasopressin (antidiuretic hormone) is a cyclic nonapeptide with pressor effects, mediated by Ca^{2+}-mobilising V1 receptors, and antidiuretic effects mediated by adenylate cyclase coupled V2 receptors.[24][25][41] It is mitogenic to Swiss 3T3 cells.[42] Vasopressin is secreted by up to 65% of small cell lung cancers and is associated with the syndrome of dilutional hyponatraemia in these patients. The demonstration that vasopressin can stimulate Ca^{2+} mobilisation in small cell lung cancer cell lines drew attention to it as a possible growth factor.[38][43] It has now been shown to stimulate the clonal growth of small cell lung cancer in soft agar at nanomolar concentrations.[44] Vasopressin may turn out to be a more important autocrine growth factor for small cell lung cancer than the bombesin like peptides.

Gastrin and cholecystokinin These gastrointestinal hormones share a carboxy-terminal pentapeptide and bind with different

---

TABLE III Factors that stimulate cell proliferation in small cell lung cancer

Bombesin/gastrin releasing peptide/neuromedin B
Bradykinin
Cholecystokinin
Galanin
Gastrin
Insulin like growth factor I
Neurotensin
Vasopressin
?β endorphin
?haemopoietic growth factors
?testosterone
?transferrin

---

affinities to common receptors. They have trophic effects on pancreatic and gut tumour cells.[1] Ca^{2+} mobilising receptors for these peptides have been found on various small cell lung cancer cell lines.[38 43 45] Cell lines exhibiting receptors were stimulated to grow by gastrin/cholecystokinin agonists and these effects were blocked by gastrin/cholecystokinin antagonists.[44 46]

Neurotensin This 13 amino acid neuropeptide was first detected in small cell lung cancer 12 years ago.[6 47] It has recently been shown to mobilise intracellular Ca^{2+} in a subset of small cell lung cancer cells, apparently acting through its own receptors.[38 43 48] The finding that exogenous neurotensin can stimulate the clonal growth of small cell lung cancer in soft agar suggests that this peptide may also act as an autocrine or paracrine growth factor for small cell lung cancer.[44 49]

Bradykinin This nonapeptide is implicated in proteolysis, clotting, and nocioceptive neurotransmission. It is a potent mitogen for Swiss 3T3 cells.[50] Bradykinin has not been detected in small cell lung cancer but it has been found to mobilise Ca^{2+} in some cell lines, acting through specific B2 receptors.[38] Bradykinin can stimulate small cell lung cancer growth in soft agar at similar concentrations to those required for Ca^{2+} mobilisation.[44]

Galanin This 29 amino acid peptide occurs in neurones of the central and peripheral nervous systems. It has been implicated in the control of pancreatic hormone release, smooth muscle contraction and neuronal excitation. It has not yet been found in small cell lung cancer. It was, however, found to mobilise intracellular Ca^{2+} in three of five small cell lung cancer cell lines tested.[38] Further studies have confirmed its ability to induce Ca^{2+} mobilisation and the formation of inositol phosphates in some small cell lung cancer cell lines. Remarkably, it stimulates clonal growth in soft agar of small cell lung cancer cells which express galanin receptors.[51]

Opioids The opioid peptides, including enkephalins, dynorphins, and endorphins, are widely distributed in the mammalian central nervous system. Several receptor subtypes have been identified chemically and pharmacologically. Two small cell lung cancer cell lines have been shown to contain opioid peptides and receptors, but whether this is a common finding in fresh tumour samples is unclear.[52] Opioids have been reported as stimulating and inhibiting clonal growth of small cell lung cancer in soft agar[49 53]; naloxone also elicits both responses.

Insulin like growth factor I

Insulin like growth factor I (IGF-I, somatomedin C) is a 70 amino acid peptide closely related to insulin and to IGF-II, with distinct high affinity receptors that have tyrosine kinase activity. Circulating concentrations of insulin like growth factor are some 1000 times higher than those of insulin, but most is complexed with specific binding proteins. Early studies of the nutritional requirements of small cell lung cancer in serum free medium established that insulin supplements were necessary,[40] but, as supraphysiological concentrations were needed for optimal growth, insulin seems likely to be acting with low affinity at the IGF-I receptor.

IGF-I is mitogenic for various cell types. It is secreted by small cell and non-small cell lung tumours and cell lines. Specific, high affinity IGF-I binding sites have been found on small cell lung cancer cells and exogenous IGF-I is mitogenic for these cells.[54–56] A monoclonal antibody to the IGF-I receptor (αIR-3) inhibited IGF-I and insulin stimulated growth of small cell lung cancer cell lines,[57] providing further evidence for an autocrine role for IGF-I. More recently, small cell lung cancer cells have been shown to secrete IGF binding proteins, which may also be important mediators of tumour growth.[58–60]

Transferrin Transferrin, an 80 kilodalton β globulin, is synthesised in the liver and transports iron in the plasma. It is required for serum free culture of small cell lung cancer[40] and is reported to be secreted by some small cell lung cancer cell lines.[61 62] Whether transferrin has a simple nutritional role or acts as an autocrine growth factor in small cell lung cancer is not clear.

Androgens In many clinical studies of small cell lung cancer men have had a worse outcome than women. This observation led to the intriguing suggestion that androgens may promote the growth of small cell lung cancer. Maasberg et al[63] found specific androgen binding in eight of 13 small cell lung cancer lines and showed that testosterone and dehydrotestosterone stimulated their growth. These growth promoting effects were blocked by cyproterone acetate and flutamide. Clinical studies with antiandrogens are now in progress.

Haemopoietic growth factors The use of harmopoietic growth factors to permit more intensive chemotherapy in patients with small cell lung cancer has led to an examination of the growth promoting activity of these factors in small cell lung cancer cells. Granulocyte colony stimulating factor (G-CSF) may be secreted by some small cell lung cancers.[64] G-CSF and granulocyte-macrophage CSF (GM-CSF) appear to bind to a minority of small cell lung cancer cell lines and can stimulate their growth in vitro.[65-67] More recently, the finding that stem cell factor and its receptor (encoded by the proto-oncogene c–*kit*) are expressed in some small cell lung cancers has fuelled speculation about the possible risks of using haemopoietic growth factors in patients with small cell lung cancer.[68-70] These effects seem unlikely to prove important clinically, but this can be tested only in large randomised trials.

Growth inhibitory factors

The identification of diverse growth promoting factors was soon followed by the finding that their actions were context dependent and that some could promote and inhibit growth under different conditions.[71] Some factors are predominantly growth inhibiting, and combinations of factors are likely to maintain homeostasis in normal tissues. This balance may be disturbed in wounds and tumours. The use of growth inhibitory factors to treat cancer is an attractive proposition. Interferons have been shown to have some growth retarding effects in small cell lung cancer and are undergoing clinical trials.[72 73]

Physalaemin This amphibian tachykinin has been identified in some small cell lung cancer cells.[74] Although specific physalaemin receptors have not been found, physalaemin mobilises intracellular Ca^{2+} in some small cell lung cancer cell lines.[75] Exogenous physalaemin inhibits clonal and mass culture growth of small cell lung cancer in vitro at picomolar concentrations, and may therefore act as an autocrine or paracrine growth regulator in vivo.[76]

Somatostatin Physiological release of somatomedins, including IGF-I, is stimulated by human growth hormone and inhibited by somatostatin. Somatostatin also has direct antiproliferative effects in many tumour types. Receptors for somatostatin are present on perhaps half of primary small cell lung cancer tumours and present an interesting target for treatment.[71 78] Long acting somatostatin analogues are now available for clinical study. The finding that somatuline can inhibit the growth of small cell lung cancer in vitro and in xenografts in nude mice has encouraged clinical studies.[79 80]

Non-small cell lung cancer

Non-small cell lung cancers form a heterogeneous group of tumours that include large cell and squamous cell carcinomas and adenocarcinomas. They show varying degrees of differentiation and can express a range of growth factors.

Epidermal growth factor and transforming growth factor α (TGF α) have been demonstrated in non-small cell cancer cell lines and tumours. Both bind to the epidermal growth factor receptor, which is present in some non-small cell lung cancers, and autocrine growth stimulation has been suggested.[81–84] p185^{neu}, the product of the HER2/neu oncogene, is a transmembrane protein having homology with the epidermal growth factor receptor and is also present in some non-small cell lung cancers.[85] Further growth factors and neuroendocrine markers expressed by non-small cell lung cancers include platelet derived growth factor, bombesin/gastrin releasing peptide, neurone specific enolase, and chromogranin A. The expression of growth factors and their receptors in some non-small cell lung cancers appears to be related to aggressive clinical behaviour and increased likelihood of response to chemotherapy.[86–88]

Therapeutic implications

The rapid progress achieved in identifying growth factors for lung cancer has raised hopes of more rational anticancer treatments. These may break the loop of autocrine or paracrine growth stimulation at the level of growth factor, receptor, or intracellular signals. The increasing evidence that multiple growth factors stimulate proliferation of these tumours suggests that no single antiproliferative agent is likely to be curative. On the other hand, the interdependence of diverse growth factors may mean that small changes in the hormonal milieu could have profound effects on growth. This approach has been exploited to good effect in the hormonal treatment of breast cancer.

The expression of growth factor receptors on cancer cells can be exploited by conjugating toxins or radioisotopes to the ligand. The epidermal growth factor receptor has been targeted in this way by conjugating *Pseudomonas* exotoxin subunits to transforming growth factor-α. The resulting compound is cytotoxic in vitro to cells carrying the epidermal growth factor receptor and cytostatic for xenografts of these tumours. Unfortunately, dose limiting toxicity occurs in normal liver and prevents therapeutic doses from being given. Further developments are needed before clinical studies can start.

Antibodies to growth factors and their receptors can be used to block autocrine or paracrine growth stimulation. The monoclonal bombesin antibody 2A11[11] has entered clinical study in patients with small cell lung cancer in the United States, at the National Cancer Institute, Bethesda, Maryland.[89] Radioisotope labelled antibody has shown some degree of localisation in the tumour and the gastrointestinal tract, and one clinical response has been seen.[90] The potential problems of anti-idiotype reactions have not been seen. To reduce this risk newer approaches, using Fab fragments and humanised antibodies (rodent antibody variable regions linked to human constant regions), are being developed.

The large size of antibodies might restrict their penetration of tumours. Small peptides are an attractive alternative approach. Like agonists or antibodies, antagonists could be linked to toxins or radioisotopes if desired. The development of peptide antagonists to neuropeptide growth factors for small cell lung cancer is an area of active research.[91] Swiss 3T3 cells have again proved useful as a model system for testing new compounds. Ligand specific antagonists, such as the pseudopeptide analogues of bombesin, have been shown to inhibit bombesin stimulated mitogenesis in these cells, and have been tested in small cell lung cancer in vitro and in vivo.[92–96] Because bombesin/gastrin releasing peptide is not mitogenic for all small cell lung cancers, specific antagonists will be useful for only a minority of patients. In contrast, broad spectrum antagonists, with activity against many mitogenic neuropeptides, will have wider application.[95 96] New peptide antagonists with enhanced potency and reduced toxicity are being developed, but much interest has also centred on the benzodiazepine-like non-peptide antagonists.[91 97] These compounds are orally bioavailable and have a longer plasma half life than the peptide antagonists.

61

The use of growth inhibitory factors as therapeutic agents is a direct development from growth factor research. Studies with somatostatin analogues have shown promise in vitro, but the results of an early clinical trial produced negative results.[98][99] The role of cytokines, such as interferon, in altering the expression of growth factors and their receptors on tumour cells is also being investigated. A study in which natural α-interferon was used as maintenance treatment in patients with small cell lung cancer in complete remission showed prolonged survival with limited disease in those receiving interferon. These results are encouraging, but need confirmation.[73] The mechanism underlying these effects remains to be determined.[72]

Increasing knowledge of the signal transduction pathways for growth factors has led to speculation that they could offer novel targets for anticancer treatment. The protein kinase C activator bryostatin is already under clinical study in Britain.[100] G proteins and oncogenes are attractive targets, as they are often overexpressed in malignant cells. The problems of delivering therapeutic agents, such as antisense oligonucleotides, into the intact cell offer further challenges to ingenuity. These approaches have the advantage of blocking signals from many mitogens. Attacking such ubiquitous targets might be expected to have toxic effects throughout the body, but this should not be assumed. The calcium channel blockers, including nifedipine and verapamil, show that selective pharmacological effects can be obtained with such apparently blunt instruments.

Studies of the expression of growth factor receptors have shown that some receptors become down–regulated after prolonged exposure to ligand (homologous desensitisation), and others are down-regulated by exposure of the cell to other ligands (heterologous desensitisation). The down–regulation of the bombesin/gastrin releasing peptide receptor after exposure of Swiss 3T3 cells to vasopressin is a good example of this.[34] This phenomenon might be exploited therapeutically by the use of partial agonists to desensitise tumour cells to growth factors.

Conclusion

Small cell lung cancer is exquisitely chemosensitive and drug treatment can reduce tumour mass dramatically but relapse due to development of resistance is almost invariable. Recent discoveries in lung tumour biology have raised hopes of new treatments and improved survival for patients with both small cell and non-small cell lung cancer.

As knowledge of the action of growth factors in lung cancer has increased, an initially simple picture has become more complex. The number of factors known to be implicated in the proliferation of small cell lung cancer is still rising, but it is clear that all the tumours secrete and respond to multiple growth factors. Understanding how these factors act opens up exciting new therapeutic strategies. Innovative compounds are already reaching patients, and close collaboration between laboratory and clinic will be needed to exploit their promise to the full.

1 Woll PJ. Neuropeptide growth factors and cancer. *Br J Cancer* 1991;**63**:469–75.

2 Ghatei MA, Sheppard MN, Henzen-Logman S, Blank MA, Polak JM, Bloom SR. Bombesin and vasoactive intestinal peptide in the developing lung: marked changes in the respiratory distress syndrome. *J Clin Endocrinol Metab* 1983;**57**:1226–32.

3 Spindel ER, Sunday ME, Hofler H, Wolfe HJ, Habener JF, Chin WW. Transient elevation of messenger RNA encoding gastrin-releasing peptide, a putative pulmonary growth factor in human fetal lung. *J Clin Invest* 1987;**80**:1172–9.

4 Moody TW, Pert CB, Gazdar AF, Carney DN, Minna JD. High levels of intracellular bombesin characterize human small cell lung cancer. *Science* 1981;**214**:1246–8.

5 Suzuki M, Yamaguchi K, Abe K, *et al.* Detection of gastrin-releasing peptide mRNA in small cell lung carcinomas and medullary thyroid carcinomas using synthetic oligodeoxy-ribo-nucleotide probes. *Jpn J Clin Oncol* 1987;**17**:157–63.

6 Wood SM, Wood JR, Ghatei MA, Lee YC, O'Shaughnessy D, Bloom SR. Bombesin, somatostatin and neurotensin-like immunoreactivity in bronchial carcinoma. *J Clin Endocrinol Metab* 1981;**53**:1310–12.

7 Rozengurt E, Sinnett-Smith J. Bombesin stimulation of DNA synthesis and cell division in cultures of Swiss 3T3 cells. *Proc Natl Acad Sci USA* 1983;**80**:2936–40.

8 Moody TW, Carney DN, Cuttitta F, Quattrocchi K, Minna JD. High affinity receptors for bombesin/GRP-like peptides on human small cell lung cancer. *Life Sci* 1985;**37**:105–13.

9 Carney DN, Cuttitta F, Moody TW, Minna JD. Selective stimulation of small cell lung cancer clonal growth by bombesin and gastrin-releasing peptide. *Cancer Res* 1987;**47**:821–5.

10 Alexander RW, Upp JR, Poston GJ, Gupta V, Townsend CM, Thompson JC. Effects of bombesin on growth of human small cell lung carcinoma in vivo. *Cancer Res* 1988;**48**:1439–41.

11 Cuttitta F, Carney DN, Mulshine J, *et al.* Bombesin-like peptides can function as autocrine growth factors in human small-cell lung carcinoma. *Nature* 1985;**316**:823–6.

12 Rozengurt E, Fabregat I, Coffer A, Gil J, Sinnett-Smith J. Mitogenic signalling through the bombesin receptor: role of a guanine nucleotide regulatory protein. *J Cell Sci* 1990;**suppl 13**:43–56.

13 Zachary I, Rozengurt E. High-affinity receptors for peptides of the bombesin family in Swiss 3T3 cells. *Proc Natl Acad Sci USA* 1985;**82**:7616–20.

14 Kris RM, Hazan R, Villines J, Moody TW, Schlessinger J. Identification of the bombesin receptor on murine and human cells by cross-linking experiments. *J Biol Chem* 1987;**262**:11215–20.

15 Zachary I, Rozengurt E. Identification of a receptor for peptides of the bombesin family in Swiss 3T3 cells by affinity cross-linking. *J Biol Chem* 1987;**262**:3947–50.

16 Sinnett-Smith J, Zachary I, Rozengurt E. Characterization of a bombesin receptor on Swiss mouse 3T3 cells by affinity cross-linking. *J Cell Biochem* 1988;**38**:237–49.

17 Spindel ER, Giladi E, Brehm P, Goodman RH, Segerson TP. Cloning and functional characterization of a complementary DNA encoding the murine fibroblast bombesin/gastrin-releasing peptide receptor. *Mol Endocrinol* 1990;4:1956–63.

18 Battey JF, Way JM, Corjay MH, *et al.* Molecular cloning of the bombesin/gastrin-releasing peptide receptor from Swiss 3T3 cells. *Proc Natl Acad Sci USA* 1991;88:395–9.

19 Battey J, Wada E. Two distinct receptor subtypes for mammalian bombesin-like peptides. *Trends Neuro Sci* 1991;14:524–8.

20 Dohlman HG, Thorner J, Caron MG, Lefkowitz RJ. Model systems for the study of seven transmembrane segment receptors. *Annu Rev Biochem* 1991;60:653–88.

21 O'Dowd BF, Lefkowitz RJ, Caron MG. Structure of the adrenergic and related receptors. *Annu Rev Neurosci* 1989;12:67–83.

22 McEachern AE, Shelton ER, Bhakta S, *et al.* Expression cloning of a rat B_2 bradykinin receptor. *Proc Natl Acad Sci USA* 1991;88:7724–8.

23 Takeda Y, Chou KB, Takeda J, Sachais BS, Krause JE. Molecular cloning, structural characterization and functional expression of the human substance P receptor. *Biochem Biophys Res Commun* 1991;179:1232–40.

24 Birnbaumer M, Siebold A, Gilbert S, *et al.* Molecular cloning of the receptor for human antidiuretic hormone. *Nature* 1992;357:333–5.

25 Lolait SJ, O'Carroll A-M, McBride OW, Konig M, Morel A, Brownstein MJ. Cloning and characterization of a vasopressin V2 receptor and possible link to nephrogenic diabetes insipidus. *Nature* 1992;357:336–9.

26 Jackson TR, Blair LAC, Marshall J, Goedert M, Hanley MR. The *mas* oncogene encodes an angiotensin receptor. *Nature* 1988;335:437–40.

27 Julius D, Livelli TJ, Jessell TM, Axel R. Ectopic expression of the serotonin 1c receptor and the triggering of malignant transformation. *Science* 1989;244:1057–62.

28 Mendoza SA, Schneider JA, Lopez-Rivas A, Sinnett-Smith JW, Rozengurt E. Early events elicited by bombesin and structurally-related peptides in quiescent Swiss 3T3 cells. II. Changes in Na^+ and Ca^{2+} fluxes, Na^+/K^+ pump activity, and intracellular pH. *J Cell Biol* 1986;102:2223–33.

29 Nishizuka Y. Intracellular signaling by hydrolysis of phospholipids and activation of protein kinase C. *Science* 1992;258:607–14.

30 Zachary I, Sinnett-Smith JW, Rozengurt E. Early events elicited by peptides of the bombesin family in Swiss 3T3 cells. I. Activation of protein kinase C and inhibition of epidermal growth factor binding. *J Cell Biol* 1986;102:2211–22.

31 Erusalimsky JD, Brooks SF, Herget T, Morris C, Rozengurt E. Molecular cloning and characterization of the acidic 80 kDa protein kinase C substrate from rat brain. *J Biol Chem* 1991;266:7073–80.

32 Zachary I, Gil J, Lehmann W, Sinnett-Smith J, Rozengurt E. Bombesin, vasopressin, and endothelin rapidly stimulate tyrosine phosphorylation in intact Swiss 3T3 cells. *Proc Natl Acad Sci USA* 1991;88:4577–81.

33 Rozengurt E. Neuropeptides as cellular growth factors: role of multiple signalling pathways. *Eur J Clin Invest* 1991;21:123–34.

34 Millar JBA, Rozengurt E. Arachidonic acid release by bombesin: a novel post-receptor target for heterologous mitogenic desensitization. *J Biol Chem* 1990;265:19973–9.

35 Rozengurt E, Sinnett-Smith J. Early signals underlying the induction of the c-*fos* and c-*myc* genes in quiescent fibroblasts: studies with bombesin and other growth factors. *Progr Nucleic Acids Res Mol Biol* 1988;35:261–95.

36 Heikkila R, Trepel JB, Cuttitta F, Neckers LM, Sausville EA. Bombesin-related peptides induce calcium mobilization in a subset of human small cell lung cancer cell lines. *J Biol Chem* 1987;262:16456–60.

37 Trepel JB, Moyer JD, Heikkila R, Sausville EA. Modulation of bombesin-induced phosphatidylinositol hydrolysis in a small-cell lung-cancer cell line. *Biochem J* 1988;255:403–10.

38 Woll PJ, Rozengurt E. Multiple neuropeptides mobilise calcium in small cell lung cancer: effects of vasopressin, bradykinin, cholecystokinin, galanin and neurotensin. *Biochem Biophys Res Commun* 1989;164:66–73.

39 Bepler G, Rotsch M, Jaques G, *et al.* Peptides and growth factors in small cell lung cancer: production, binding sites, and growth effects. *J Cancer Res Clin Oncol* 1988;114:235–44.

40 Simms E, Gazdar AF, Abrams PG, Minna JD. Growth of human small cell (oat cell) carcinoma of the lung in serum-free growth factor-supplemented medium. *Cancer Res* 1980;40:4356–63.

41 Morel A, O'Carroll A-M, Brownstein MJ, Lolait SJ. Molecular cloning and expression of a rat V1a arginine vasopressin receptor. *Nature* 1992;**356**:523–6.

42 Rozengurt E, Legg A, Pettican P. Vasopressin stimulation of mouse 3T3 cell growth. *Proc Natl Acad Sci USA* 1979;**76**:1284–7.

43 Bunn PA, Dienhart DG, Chan D, *et al*. Neuropeptide stimulation of calcium flux in human lung cancer cells: delineation of alternate pathways. *Proc Natl Acad Sci USA* 1990;**87**:2162–6.

44 Sethi T, Rozengurt E. Multiple neuropeptides stimulate clonal growth of small cell lung cancer: effects of bradykinin, vasopressin, cholecystokinin, galanin and neurotensin. *Cancer Res* 1991;**51**:3621–3.

45 Staley J, Fiskum G, Moody TW. Cholecystokinin elevates cytosolic calcium in small cell lung cancer cells. *Biochem Biophys Res Commun* 1989;**163**:605–10.

46 Sethi T, Rozengurt E. Gastrin stimulates Ca^{2+} mobilization and clonal growth in small cell lung cancer cells. *Cancer Res* 1992;**52**:6031–5.

47 Goedert M, Reeve JG, Emson PC, Bleehen NM. Neurotensin in human small cell lung carcinoma. *Br J Cancer* 1984;**50**:179–83.

48 Staley J, Fiskum G, Davis TP, Moody TW. Neurotensin elevates cytosolic calcium in small cell lung cancer cells. *Peptides* 1989;**10**:1217–21.

49 Davis TP, Burgess HS, Crowell S, Moody TW, Culling-Berglund A, Liu RH. β-endorphin and neurotensin stimulate in vitro clonal growth of human SCLC cells. *Eur J Pharmacol* 1989;**161**:283–5.

50 Woll PJ, Rozengurt E. Two classes of antagonist interact with receptors for the mitogenic neuropeptides bombesin, bradykinin and vasopressin. *Growth Factors* 1988;**1**:75–83.

51 Sethi T, Rozengurt E. Galanin stimulates Ca^{2+} mobilization, inositol phosphate accumulation and clonal growth in small cell lung cancer cell lung cancer cells. *Cancer Res* 1991;**51**:1674–9.

52 Roth KA, Barchas JD. Small cell carcinoma cell lines contain opioid peptides and receptors. *Cancer* 1986;**57**:769–73.

53 Maneckjee R, Minna JD. Opioid and nicotine receptors affect growth regulation of human lung cancer cell lines. *Proc Natl Acad Sci USA* 1990;**87**:3294–8.

54 Jaques G, Rotsch M, Wegmann C, Worsch U, Maasberg M, Havemann K. Production of immunoreactive insulin-like growth factor I and response to exogenous IGF-I in small cell lung cancer cell lines. *Exp Cell Res* 1988;**176**:336–43.

55 Macaulay VM, Teale JD, Everard MJ, Joshi GP, Smith IE, Millar JL. Somatomedin-C/insulin-like growth factor-I is a mitogen for human small cell lung cancer. *Br J Cancer* 1988;**57**:91–3.

56 Macaulay VM, Everard MJ, Teale JD, *et al*. Autocrine function for insulin-like growth factor I in human small cell lung cancer cell lines and fresh tumor cells. *Cancer Res* 1990;**50**:2511–17.

57 Nakanishi Y, Mulshine JL, Kasprzyk PG, *et al*. Insulin-like growth factor-I can mediate autocrine proliferation of human small cell lung cancer cell lines in vitro. *J Clin Invest* 1988;**82**:354–9.

58 Jaques G, Kiefer P, Rotsch M, *et al*. Production of insulin-like growth factor binding proteins by small-cell lung cancer cell lines. *Exp Cell Res* 1989;**184**:396–406.

59 Reeve JG, Payne JA, Bleehen NM. Production of immunoreactive insulin-like growth factor-I (IGF-I) and IGF-I binding proteins by human lung tumours. *Br J Cancer* 1990;**61**:727–31.

60 Kiefer P, Jaques G, Schöneberger J, Heinrich G, Havemann K. Insulin-like growth factor binding protein expression in human small cell lung cancer cell lines. *Exp Cell Res* 1991;**192**:414–17.

61 Nakanishi Y, Cuttitta F, Kasprzyk PG, *et al*. Growth factor effects on small cell lung cancer cells using a colorimetric assay: can a transferrin-like factor mediate autocrine growth? *Exp Cell Biol* 1988;**56**:74–85.

62 Vostrejs M, Moran PL, Seligman PA. Transferrin synthesis by small cell lung cancer cells acts as an autocrine regulator of cellular proliferation. *J Clin Invest* 1988;**82**:331–9.

63 Maasberg M, Rotsch M, Jaques G, Enderle-Schmidt U, Weehle R, Havemann K. Androgen receptors, androgen-dependent proliferation, and 5α-reductase activity of small-cell lung cancer cell lines. *Int J Cancer* 1989;**43**:685–91.

64 Abe K, Kameya T, Yamaguchi K, *et al*. Hormone-producing lung cancers. Endocrinologic and morphologic studies. In: Becker KL, Gazdar AF, eds. *The endocrine lung in health and disease*. London: WB Saunders, 1984:549–95.

65 Avalos BR, Gasson JC, Hedvat C, et al. Human granulocyte colony-stimulating factor: biologic activities and receptor characterization on hematopoietic cells and small cell lung cancer cell lines. Blood 1990;75:851–7.

66 Foulke RS, Marshall MH, Trotta PP, von Hoff DD. In vitro assessment of the effects of granulocyte–macrophage colony-stimulating factor on primary human tumors and derived lines. Cancer Res 1990;50:6264–7.

67 Vellenga E, Biesma B, Meyer C, Wagteveld L, Esselink M, de Vries EGE. The effects of five hematopoietic growth factors on human small cell lung carcinoma cell lines: interleukin 3 enhances the proliferation in one of the eleven cell lines. Cancer Res 1991;51:73–6.

68 Witte ON. Steel locus defines new multipotent growth factor. Cell 1990;63:5–6.

69 Sekido Y, Obata Y, Ueda R, et al. Preferential expression of c-kit protooncogene transcripts in small cell lung cancer. Cancer Res 1991;51:2416–19.

70 Hibi K, Takahashi T, Sekido Y, et al. Coexpression of the stem cell factor and the c-kit genes in small cell lung cancer. Oncogene 1991;6:2291–6.

71 Sporn MB, Roberts AB. Peptide growth factors are multifunctional. Nature 1988;332:217–19.

72 Jett JR. Is there a role for interferon in the treatment of small cell lung cancer? Lung Cancer 1989;5:281–6.

73 Mattson K, Niiranen A, Pyrhönen S, et al. Natural interferon alpha as maintenance therapy for small cell lung cancer. Eur J Cancer 1992;28A:1387–91.

74 Lazarus LH, DiAugustine RP, Jahnke GD, Hernandez O. Physalaemin: an amphibian tachykinin in human lung small-cell carcinoma. Science 1983;219:79–81.

75 Takuwa N, Takuwa Y, Ohue Y, et al. Stimulation of calcium mobilization but not proliferation by bombesin and tachykinin neuropeptides in human small cell lung cancer cells. Cancer Res 1990;50:240–4.

76 Bepler G, Carney DN, Gazdar AF, Minna JD. In vitro growth inhibition of human small cell lung cancer by physalaemin. Cancer Res 1987;47:2371–5.

77 Reubi JC, Waser B, Sheppard M, Macaulay V. Somatostatin receptors are present in small-cell but not in non-small-cell lung carcinomas: relationship to EGF-receptors. Int J Cancer 1990;45:269–74.

78 Sagman U, Mullen JB, Kovacs K, Kerbel R, Ginsberg R, Reubi J-C. Identification of somatostatin receptors in human small cell lung carcinoma. Cancer 1990;66:2129–33.

79 Taylor JE, Bogden AE, Moreau J-P, Coy DH. In vitro and in vivo inhibition of human small cell lung carcinoma (NCI-H69) growth by a somatostatin analogue. Biochem Biophys Res Commun 1988;153:81–6.

80 Bogden AE, Taylor JE, Moreau J-P, Coy DH, LePage DJ. Response of human lung tumor xenografts to treatment with a somatostatin analogue (somatuline). Cancer Res 1990;50:4360–5.

81 Haeder M, Rotsch M, Bepler G, et al. Epidermal growth factor receptor expression in human lung cancer cell lines. Cancer Res 1988;48:1132–6.

82 Söderdahl G, Betsholtz C, Johansson A, Nilsson K, Bergh J. Differential expression of platelet-derived growth factor and transforming growth factor genes in small- and non-small-cell human lung carcinoma lines. Int J Cancer 1988;41:636–41.

83 Veale D, Kerr N, Gibson GJ, Harris AL. Characterization of epidermal growth factor receptor in primary human non-small cell lung cancer. Cancer Res 1989;49:1313–17.

84 Tateishi M, Ishida T, Mitsudomi T, Kaneko S, Sugimachi K. Immunohistochemical evidence of autocrine growth factors in adenocarcinoma of the human lung. Cancer Res 1990;50:7077–80.

85 Kern JA, Schwartz DA, Nordberg JE, et al. p185^{neu} expression in human lung adenocarcinomas predicts shortened survival. Cancer Res 1990;50:5184–91.

86 Mooi WJ, Dewar A, Springall D, Polak JM, Addis BJ. Non-small cell lung carcinomas with neuroendocrine features. A light microscopic, immunohistochemical and ultrastructural study of 11 cases. Histopathology 1988;13:329–37.

87 Graziano SL, Mazid R, Newman N, et al. The use of neuroendocrine immunoperoxidase markers to predict chemotherapy response in patients with non-small-cell lung cancer. J Clin Oncol 1989;7:1398–406.

88 Hamid QA, Corrin B, Dewar A, Hoefler H, Sheppard MN. Expression of gastrin-releasing peptide (human bombesin) gene in large cell undifferentiated carcinoma of the lung. J Pathol 1990;161:145–51.

66

89 Avis IL, Kovacs TOG, Kasprzyk PG, et al. Preclinical evaluation of an anti-autocrine growth factor monoclonal antibody for treatment of patients with small-cell lung cancer. JNCI 1991;83:1470–6.

90 Kelley MJ, Avis I, Linnoila RI, et al. Complete response in a patient with small cell lung cancer (SCLC) treated in a phase II trial using a murine monoclonal antibody (2A11) directed against gastrin releasing peptide. Proc Am Soc Clin Oncol 1993;12:339.

91 Woll PJ, Sethi T, Rozengurt E. Neuropeptide growth factors and antagonists. In: Tritton TR, Hickman JA, eds. Cancer Chemotherapy. Oxford: Blackwell, 1993:128–45.

92 Woll PJ, Rozengurt E. [Leu[13]-psi(CH2NH)Leu[14]]bombesin is a specific bombesin receptor antagonist in Swiss 3T3 cells. Biochem Biophys Res Commun 1988;155:359–65.

93 Mahmoud S, Staley J, Taylor J, et al. [Psi[13,14]] bombesin analogues inhibit growth of small cell lung cancer in vitro and in vivo. Cancer Res 1991;51:1798–802.

94 Thomas F, Arvelo F, Antoine E, Jacrot M, Poupon MF. Antitumoral activity of bombesin analogues on small cell lung cancer xenografts: relationship with bombesin receptor expression. Cancer Res 1992;52:4872–7.

95 Woll PJ, Rozengurt E. A neuropeptide antagonist that inhibits the growth of small cell lung cancer in vitro. Cancer Res 1990;50:3968–73.

96 Langdon S, Sethi T, Ritchie A, Muir M, Smyth J, Rozengurt E. Broad spectrum neuropeptide antagonists inhibit the growth of small cell lung cancer in vivo. Cancer Res 1992;52:4554–7.

97 Chang RSL, Lotti VJ. Biochemical and pharmacological characterization of an extremely potent and selective non-peptide cholecystokinin antagonist. Proc Natl Acad Sci USA 1986;83:4923–6.

98 Taylor JE, Moreau J-P, Baptiste L, Moody TW. Octapeptide analogues of somatostatin inhibit the clonal growth and vasoactive intestinal peptide-stimulated cyclic AMP formation in human small cell lung cancer cells. Peptides 1991;12:839–43.

99 Macaulay VM, Smith IE, Everard MJ, Teale JD, Reubi J-C, Millar JL. Experimental and clinical studies with somatostatin analogue octreotide in small cell lung cancer. Br J Cancer 1991;64:451–6.

100 Prendiville J, Crowther D, Thatcher N, et al. A phase I study of intravenous bryostatin I in patients with advanced cancer. Br J Cancer 1993;68:418–24.

5 The antigens of lung cancer

ROBERT L SOUHAMI

The growth of interest in the biology of lung cancer is a welcome product of frustration with the results of current treatment. The past 15 years have seen a considerable increase in our knowledge of the disease, and we can but hope that therapeutic advances will ensue. It is the most common cause of death from cancer in men, and in the United States in the past two years it has overtaken breast cancer as the most common cause of fatal cancer in women. An additional spur to biological investigation has been the recognition of four pathological types of the disease. There is growing acceptance of the hypothesis that lung cancer starts in a cell capable of differentiating into various pathological forms (figure 1). This is supported by the occurrence of mixed pathological types (for example, mixed squamous and small cell). In cell lines and in biopsy material it has been shown that neuroendocrine features, typical of small cell lung cancer, can be found in adenocarcinoma

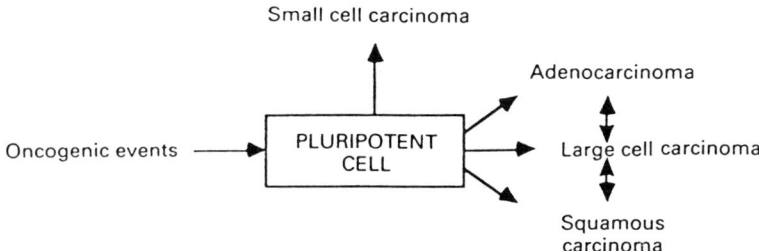

Figure 1   Hypothesis for the development of histological types of lung cancer.

and that cytokeratins, which are uniformly found in squamous cell carcinomas, are expressed in small cell lung cancer.

Small cell lung cancer shows the typical pathological features of neuroendocrine differentiation: neurosecretory dense core granules, chromogranin A, cytoplasmic L dopa decarboxylase, the glycolytic enzyme neurone specific enolase, and production of hormones and neuropeptides. There is some evidence that when some of these features are detected in an adenocarcinoma it is more likely to respond to chemotherapy,[1] though more recent studies have indicated that the effect is small.[2]

These considerations indicate that the antigens detected in lung cancer are likely to be expressed, in some degree, in all pathological types and will be representative of antigens found in neuroendocrine,[3] squamous, and glandular tissues, and in carcinomas at other sites. Some of these antigens are potential targets for antibody directed treatment. They are molecules that are associated with a wide range of functions of normal fetal and malignant cells. Strictly speaking, they are not "tumour antigens" (though they are sometimes referred to as such) because they are not tumour specific in the sense of appearing only on tumour cells. Monoclonal antibodies, produced by somatic cell hybridisation, have led to the definition of a wide range of cellular antigens, many of them proteins whose function has now been well characterised and whose amino acid sequences have been determined. They are broadly categorised as cell-cell attachment molecules, antigens binding to extracellular matrix proteins, antigens that are receptors for transmembrane signal induction, and blood group antigens.

Types of cellular antigens

Cell-cell attachment molecules

Carcinoembryonic antigens are a family of proteins closely related to the immunoglobulin gene "superfamily."[4] Carcinoembryonic antigens are expressed during fetal life and re-expressed in various neoplasms, typically in adenocarcinomas. Other members of this "superfamily" include the neural cell adhesion molecule, and recent workshops on lung cancer antigens have shown that this is expressed in most small cell lung cancer lines and biopsy specimens, and appears to be an important marker of the neuro-endocrine phenotype. Carcinoembryonic antigens are also

69

expressed in small cell lung cancer and other forms of lung cancer and may be associated with an adverse prognosis.[25] The neural cell adhesion molecule (NCAM) is a cell-cell attachment protein that is heavily glycosylated. It exists in several major isoforms. There are two transmembrane linked forms, a truncated form attached to membrane phospholipid (via glycosylphosphatidylinositol) and a soluble form in muscle and brain. The genetic basis for this variation lies in alternative splicing of the gene for the neural cell adhesion molecule.[6] The predominant form of NCAM in small cell lung cancer cell lines is the transmembrane 140 kilodalton molecule.[7] The molecule has the property of homophilic binding (figure 2). The degree of binding is inversely related to the amount of glycosylation. Heavily glycosylated NCAM is a feature of small cell lung cancer; less glycosylation is found in carcinoid tumours. A heavily glycosylated form has been described in Wilms' tumours. The forms of NCAM expressed in small cell lung cancer have not yet been systematically analysed. Many monoclonal antibodies have been made to NCAM and many seem to recognise a relatively restricted region of the peptide backbone.

Other carcinoembryonic antigen like molecules are myelin associated glycoprotein and an antigen found on melanoma cells.[8] A surface glycoprotein of molecular weight 40 kilodaltons was found, in the lung cancer workshops, to be expressed on lung cancers and a wide range of epithelia and epithelial malignancies. The gene has been cloned[9] and seems to be closely related to an extracellular matrix protein, nidogen. Other cell attachment molecules, such as the intercellular adhesion molecule, are expressed on melanoma

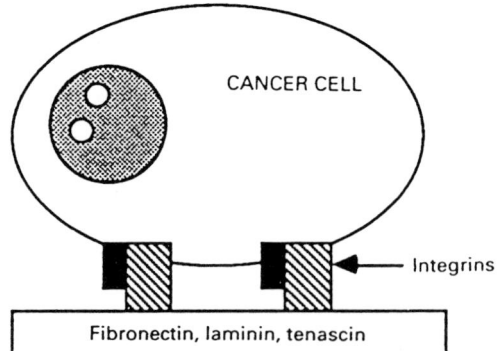

Figure 2   Binding of integrins to extracellular matrix proteins.

and other cancer cells. The class I histocompatibility antigens are found on all forms of lung cancer, but class II is poorly expressed on small cell lung cancers, though its presence can be induced by treatment with interferon α.

Antigens that bind to extracellular matrix proteins

Many tumour cells both secrete and have receptors for extracellular matrix proteins (figure 3). Proteins such as collagen, fibronectin, lamina, and tenascin are essential components of the extracellular matrix. Integrins are heterodimeric transmembrane receptor proteins that bind to laminin, collagen, and fibronectin. In doing so they link the cytoskeleton of the cell with the matrix.[10] The integrin family is a complex in which the α chain varies and the β peptide defines the class. The variety of integrin expression is apparently reduced in cancer. Integrins appear in a later stage of cellular differentiation and are found on squamous cancers. Glycolipid antigens (GD_2 and GD_3) are also expressed in lung cancer and may be important in cell invasion in this and other tumours.[11]

Antigens that are receptors concerned with transmembrane signal induction

The cell membrane contains a range of receptors for growth factors, cytokines, and toxins as well as proteins concerned with drug attachment and efflux. Figure 4 shows some of these proteins and indicates some of the diversity of function. The epidermal

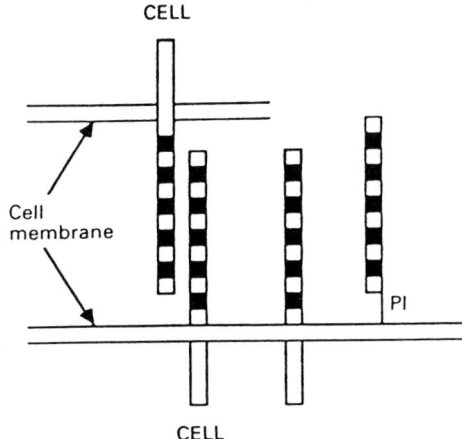

Figure 3   Major isoforms of neural cell adhesion molecule showing homophilic binding. The dark regions indicate repetitive domains. PI—phosphotidylinositol linked form. A form of NCAM is also synthesised that is detached from the cytoplasmic membrane.

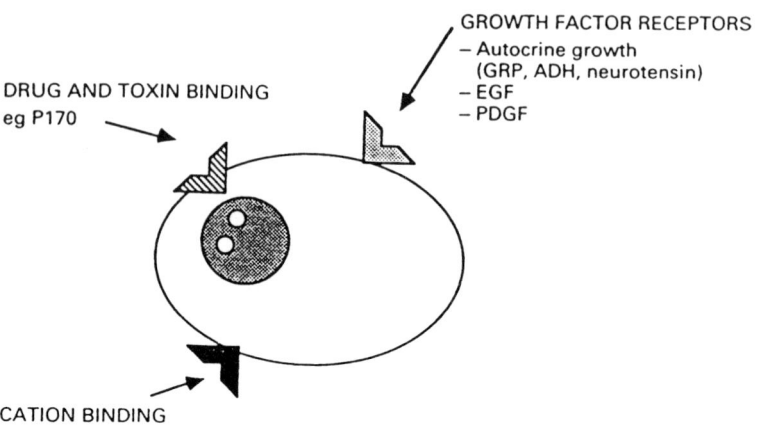

Figure 4   Some membrane receptor molecules, recognised by monoclonal antibodies, on the lung cancer cell. GRP—gastrin releasing peptide; ADH—antidiuretic hormone; EGF—epidermal growth factor; PDGF—platelet derived growth factor.

growth factor receptor (EGFR) is expressed on non-small cell lung cancer and is associated with an adverse prognosis. Receptors for insulin like growth factors have been shown on small cell lung cancer cells. These receptors and others, such as those for platelet derived growth factor, are widely distributed on tumours and normal cells. Of particular interest in small cell lung cancer is the expression of receptors for growth inducing peptides, such as gastrin releasing peptide (bombesin), which are secreted by the tumour and which, on becoming bound to the tumour cell, promote cell division—that is, autocrine growth stimulation.

Other membrane associated proteins concern cellular functions of detoxification and cation transport. The p170 glycoprotein is associated with cellular resistance to the effects of naturally occurring antitumour substances, such as doxorubicin, epipodophyllotoxin, and colchicine. The protein acts as a drug efflux mechanism and methods to circumvent its action may yet give useful therapeutic results. MBrl is a glycosphingolipid expressed on breast and lung cancer cells whose function is not clear.

Membrane receptors taking part in the transport of calcium, iron, copper, and other cations are found on the surface of lung cancer cells (and other tumour cells) as on normal cells and other tumours. Up–regulation or altered expression of these receptors has not yet been described in lung cancer.

Blood group antigens

Carbohydrate antigens on glycolipids are strongly expressed on many epithelial tumours.[11] Many of these are blood group antigens such as Lewis[x] and Lewis[y], and some are expressed less (or not at all) on the normal epithelium from which the tumour is derived. In this sense they sometimes represent oncofetal antigens, which may be expressed transiently during tissue development and are re-expressed in neoplasia.

Some of these carbohydrate antigens are also found on glycoproteins, such as mucins or adhesion molecules, and the patterns of glycosylation in these high molecular weight structures may be different in normal and malignant cells. Blood group and glycolipid antigens are expressed on both small cell and non-small cell lung cancers.[12] The presence of glycosylated H antigen H/Le[y]/Le[b] is associated with worse prognosis in surgically resected non-small cell lung cancer.[13]

Lung cancer antigen workshops

Two recent workshops[14 15] have been undertaken to attempt to introduce a taxonomic description of the antigens being recognised by the numerous monoclonal antibodies to lung cancer cells. A summary of the major clusters of reactivity is given in table I. Cluster 1 is NCAM[16] and there are now numerous examples of monoclonal antibodies that react with this molecule. Many of them cross block, indicating recognition of a common epitope, but some do not. They appear to recognise protein rather than sugar residues. Cluster 2 is the gp40 glycoprotein described previously. Clusters W6 and W8 are blood group haptens, and W7 is a high molecular weight mucin. Clusters 4 and 5 are extremely interesting glycoproteins with both neural and epithelial reactivity found on small cell lung cancer cells and of unknown function. The workshops showed that neuroendocrine differentiation was a much more pronounced feature of small cell lung cancer than of non-small cell lung cancer, but that overlap of neuroendocrine and epithelial features occurred.

TABLE I   Lung cancer antigen classification based on the analysis of the Second Lung Cancer Antigen Workshop*

Cluster	Monoclonal antibodies	Comments
1	RNL1, MOC-1, MOC-191, NCC-LU-243, NCC-LU-246, SEN 6, SEN 36, NE 150, S-L 11·14, NE 25 (also UJ13A, ERIC-1 from other sources)	Neural cell adhesion molecule.[10] Evidence for different epitopes. Form of molecule on SCLC not known. Distribution: SCLC, carcinoid, renal carcinoma, neuroblastoma, nerve, muscle, thyroid epithelium
2	MOC-31, MOC-38, MOC-151, MOC-181, AUA 1, S-L 2·21, probably PE-35 and S-L 4·20	40 kDa transmembrane glycoprotein gene is cloned.[12] Efficient in immunotoxin mediated cytotoxicity. Distribution: SCLC, carcinoid, normal and malignant epithelium
w4	SWA 21, SWA 22, probably SWA 11	Glycosylated protein 45 kDa. Distribution: SCLC, neuroblastoma, carcinoid, adenocarcinoma and squamous carcinoma, renal tubules, granulocytes
5	SWA 4, SWA 23, LAM 8	Antigens of 90–135 and 200 kDa, probably sialoglycoproteins. Distribution: SCLC, carcinoid adenocarcinomas, weakly with squamous carcinomas, nerve, renal tubules
5A	SWA 20, probably SEN 3 and SEN 31	Antigens of 40, 100, 180 kDa sialoglycoproteins. Distribution: similar to cluster 5
w6	MOV 15, NCC-ST-433, probably NCC-LU-152	Le^y. Distribution: broad epithelial reactivity
w7	NCC-ST-439, NCC-CO-450	High molecular weight mucins. Distribution: broad epithelial reactivity
w8	A-80, NCC-LU-35, NCC-LU-81	Blood group A trisaccharide. Distribution: broad epithelial reactivity

*Fifty one of 87 monoclonal antibodies were not assigned to a cluster, so this is in no sense a complete description of the antigens to which monoclonal antibodies have been made.
SCLC—small cell lung cancer.

Clinical approaches using cell surface antigens

Clinical interest in these antigens comes from their potential use as targets for antibody directed treatment (figure 5). Such treat-

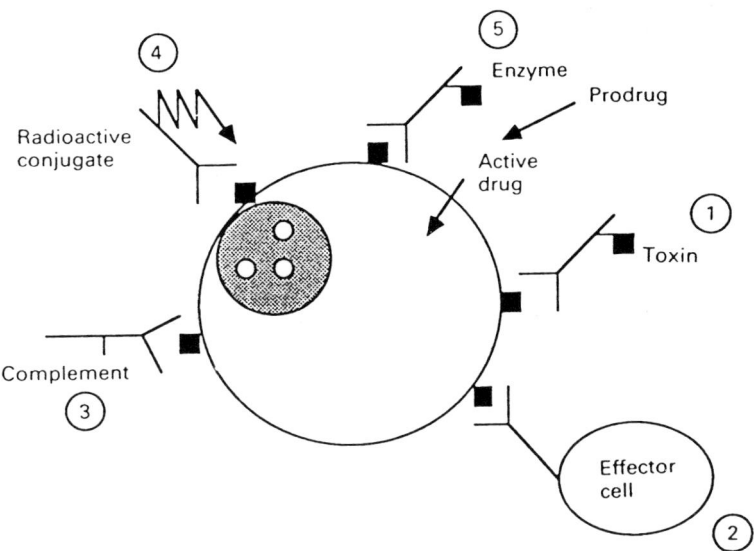

Figure 5 Potential mechanisms for tumour cell killing by monoclonal reagents. 1: a toxin is coupled to antibody that is internalised, resulting in toxin mediated cell death; 2: the antibody acts as a bridge to a cytolytic effector cell; 3: the antibody induces complement mediated lysis; 4: the antibody is conjugated to a radionuclide that irradiates the tumour; 5: the antibody is conjugated to an enzyme that activates an inert prodrug in the region of the tumour (or normal tissue).

ment might be with radiolabelled antibody, where the cell and its neighbours might be killed by radiation, or by toxins (such as the ricin A chain) linked to antibody (gp40 may be especially effective at internalising bound antibody), or by more complex methods, such as the use of a prodrug administered with an antibody coupled to an enzyme, which converts the prodrug to a cytotoxic form only at the site at which the antibody-enzyme conjugate is bound (that is, the tumour). Other approaches use antibodies that lyse cells in the presence of complement or allow cell killing by effector cells such as activated cytotoxic T cells. Phase I clinical trials using these approaches are now beginning.

Some of the antigens are more promising targets than others. Ideally, the antigen should be expressed on most cells in all cases of a given type of tumour. In practice some degree of heterogeneity is always found. The antigen should be expressed on as small a number of normal tissues as possible, and especially not on those

75

that are likely to be dose limiting (bone marrow precursor cells, for example). So far there has been little evidence that antigens unique to particular tumours (and not found in normal tissues) are likely to be found, but this may not invalidate the approach. Of course, the finding on tumour cells of altered epitopes of an antigen found on normal tissues would be a step towards increased specificity, but so far there is little indication that this is likely. New methods of production of monoclonal antibodies using molecular biology may make the rather "hit or miss" approach based on hybridomas obsolete. Progress in this approach to lung cancer treatment is highly probable.

1 Graziano SL, Mazio R, Newman N, et al. The use of neuroendocrine immunoperoxidase markers to predict chemotherapy response in patients with non small cell lung cancer. J Clin Oncol 1989;7:1389–406.
2 Ruckdeschel JC, Linniola RI, Mulshine JL, et al. The impact of neuroendocrine and epithelial differentiation on response and survival in lung cancer. Proc Am Soc Clin Oncol 1991;A849.
3 Linniola RI, Mulshine JL, Steinber SM, et al. Neuroendocrine differentiation in endocrine and non-endocrine lung carcinomas. Am J Clin Pathol 1988;90:641–52.
4 Oikawa S, Imaj S, Moguchi T, et al. The carcinoembryonic antigen (CEA) contains multiple immunoglobulin-like domains. Biochem Biophys Res Commun 1987;144:634–42.
5 Linniola RI, Ruckdeschel JC, Piantadosi S, et al. The impact of neuroendocrine and epithelial differentiation on recurrence and survival in patients with resected non small cell lung cancer: the LCSG experience. Proc Am Soc Clin Oncol 1991;A850.
6 Owens GS, Edelman GM, Cunningham BA. Organisation of the neural cell adhesion molecule (N-CAM) gene: alternative exon usage as the basis for different membrane associated domains. Proc Natl Acad Sci USA 1987;84:294–8.
7 Carbone DP, Koros AMC, Linnoila RI, Jewett P, Gazdar AF. Neural cell adhesion molecule expression and messenger RNA splicing patterns in lung cancer cell lines are correlated with neuroendocrine phenotype and growth morphology. Cancer Res 1991;51:6142–9.
8 Salzer JL, Holmes WP, Colman DR. The amino acid sequences of the myelin-associated glycoproteins: homology to the immunoglobulin gene superfamily. J Cell Biol 1987;104:957–65.
9 Simon B, Podolsky DK, Moldenhhauer G, et al. Epithelial glycoprotein is a member of a family of epithelial cell surface antigens homologous to nidogen, a matrix adhesion protein. Proc Natl Acad Sci USA 1990;87:2755–9.
10 Buck CA, Horwitz AF. Cell surface receptors for extra-cellular matrix molecules. Annu Rev Cell Biol 1987;13:179–205.
11 Weiner DB, Nordbert J, Robinson R, et al. Expression of the neu gene-encoded protein (P185^{neu}) in human non small cell lung carcinomas of the lung. Cancer Res 1990;50:421–5.
12 Andrews CM, Seiler NS, Magnani JL. Detailed epitope mapping of carbohydrate antigens recognised by antibodies from the Lung Cancer Workshop. Br J Cancer 1991;63(suppl X14):36.
13 Miyake M, Taki T, Hitomi S, Hakomori S-I. Correlation of expression of H/Le^y/Le^b antigens with survival in patients with carcinoma of the lung. N Engl J Med 1992;327:14–18.
14 Souhami RL, Beverley PCL, Bobrow LG. Antigens of small cell lung cancer. First International Workshop. Lancet 1987;ii:325–6.
15 Souhami RL, Beverley PCL, Bobrow LG, Ledermann JA. Results of central data analysis: 2nd International Workshop on Small Cell Lung Cancer Antigens. JNCI 1991;83:609–12.
16 Patel K, Moore SE, Dickson G, et al. Neural cell adhesion molecule (N-CAM) is the antigen recognised by monoclonal antibodies of similar specificity in small cell lung carcinoma and neuroblastoma. Int J Cancer 1989;44:573–6.

6 How much investigation?

MARTIN F MUERS

In any field of medical practice investigations have to have a clear purpose and must benefit the patient. They must therefore answer worthwhile questions. At a time of scarce resources for health care, the doctor must ensure that the most efficient pathway is chosen—in the sense of minimising the total personal, financial, and time cost, for the maximum benefit—better length and quality of life.

For a patient in whom the possibility of lung cancer has been raised, investigations are needed to answer two such questions:

1 *Is* it lung cancer? (and what sort of lung cancer is it?)—*the diagnosis.*
2 What ought to be done about it?—*the management.*

In practice tests needed for (1) may provide some answers to (2). For clarity, they will be considered separately in the discussion that follows.

Diagnosis (figure 1)

The diagnosis of lung cancer can be made at several levels—for example, after the history and examination, after a radiograph and blood tests, after an abnormal bronchoscopy, and pathologically. It is important to recognise at the outset that the objective is to establish a diagnosis with sufficient precision for a correct management decision to be made. As the management options are increasing, so does the need for greater precision.

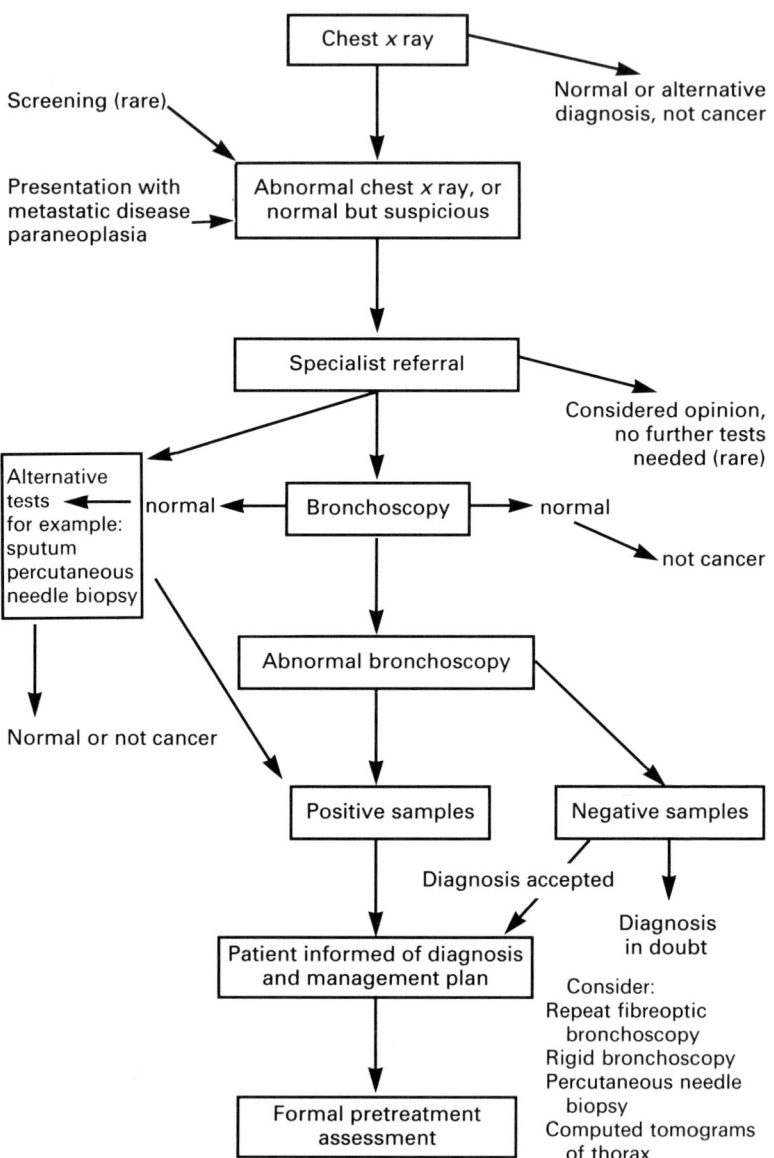

Figure 1   Investigation pathway in diagnosis of lung cancer.

It is sometimes held that a precise diagnosis is not justified because "it will not affect management". This attitude is increasingly outdated. Two aspects are relevant. The first is the question of confidence and prognosis. Firm knowledge that a person has lung cancer will allow the doctor to help the patient to come to terms with a definite diagnosis. This is always easier to manage psychologically than uncertainty.[1] Furthermore, the prognosis is then clearer and this always allows more accurate and compassionate advice to be given to the patient and family. Second, it is increasingly the case that more precise knowledge *will* lead to better tailored treatment. Examples are the advent of short course radiotherapy,[2] short course chemotherapy for small cell lung cancer,[3] laser treatment for high endobronchial lesions,[4] endobronchial radiotherapy for lower stenosing lesions,[5] and better patient selection for surgery at all ages. Because of these developments, there is now a very strong case for all patients with a possible diagnosis of lung cancer to be assessed by a specialist, such as a chest physician, oncologist, or cardiothoracic surgeon.

The average age of patients with lung cancer is rising. United Kingdom regional data from the Yorkshire Cancer Registry have shown that the mean age at diagnosis has increased from 66 to 69·5 years between 1975 and 1990.[67] The same registry study has shown that the prognosis of patients over 70 who have had surgery has improved.[6] Such treatment cannot take place unless investigations are carried out. The overall regional rate of histological verification rose from 40% to 60% over the 10 year period studied and in the over 75s from 19% to 39%.[67] Although it is probably adequate to rely on the findings of a chest radiographic mass to support a diagnosis of lung cancer in a clubbed, moribund smoker of 75 with a large liver and a hoarse voice of recent onset, in a fitter person of the same age with a different presentation, fibreoptic bronchoscopy, thoracic computed tomogram, etc, would probably be justified.

History, examination, and chest radiograph

Although the possibility of lung cancer may emerge because of a non-respiratory presentation, such as a late onset fit or hypercalcaemia, in 70% of cases it arises after a thoracic or metastatic presentation and a conventional history and examination. It is almost never appropriate to make the diagnosis and manage a patient without a radiograph and usually an accompanying lateral examination. An adequate direct access service for general practitioners should provide a report inside a week and nearly all districts have this.[8] A normal radiograph, however, does not exclude the diagnosis.[9 10] At this stage, and before any other tests are done, it is usually clear whether further investigations are warranted, having taken into account the patient's general condition and the likely prognosis. They nearly always are. The next important step is usually bronchoscopy and at the same time blood tests should be done.

Blood tests

The only tumour marker of any clinical use is neurone specific enolase (NSE). This peptide is at low concentrations in normal blood, and increased values are found in a high proportion of patients with small cell lung cancer.[11] It is not very sensitive[12] but is suggestive of the diagnosis if the clinical picture is of lung cancer—that is, specificity is relatively good. Other tumour markers such as carcinoembryonic antigen (CEA)[12] and phosphohexose isomerase (PHI)[13] are not clinically useful and although others such as (monoclonal) migration inhibitory antibody (MIA–5–5) promise better[14] there is no justification for measuring these outside research protocols.[15]

If abnormal, other blood values can raise the probability of systemic disease such as neoplasia. Examples are a high viscosity[16] or C reactive protein,[17] a low haemoglobin concentration,[16] raised alkaline phosphatase, or bilirubin, a raised calcium, or a low sodium.

Fibreoptic bronchoscopy

The development of fibreoptic bronchoscopy has revolutionised chest medicine, and technical developments and research into procedures now mean that there are very few patients who cannot have an elective examination.[18–20] The purposes of fibreoptic bronchoscopy are:

1   to confirm or reinforce a radiological diagnosis of lung cancer by seeing the lesion;
2   to obtain samples to confirm neoplasia and to type the cancer;
3   to assess operability;
4   to assess whether and in what way a patient's chest symptoms are caused by endobronchial disease.

Elective fibreoptic bronchoscopy with suitable preoperative checks[21] and attention to sedation[22][23] (or using none at all),[24] oxygenation,[25] and local anaesthesia[26][27] is now a very safe procedure. The complication rate in the 38 000 bronchoscopies reported to the British survey in 1983[28] was 0·12%, with most of these relating to inappropriate sedation. This rate and the then mortality of 0·04% are probably lower now in outpatient practice.[29] The elderly may be safely and usefully examined[30][31] and a low forced expiratory volume (FEV1)—for example, of less than 0·8 litres—requires caution and care rather than a refusal to examine.

Absolute contraindications remain a myocardial infarction within six weeks, uncorrected coagulopathies, and severe uncontrollable respiratory failure. Superior vena cava obstruction is not a contraindication. Abnormal mucosa should be sampled whenever possible. Bronchial washes (2 × 20 ml saline) should be done in the area of radiographic abnormality if no lesion is seen. Recent studies have shown that lesions should be sampled by a combination of brush or catheter for cytology and four to five forceps biopsy specimens.[32][33] There is moderately good evidence that a final wash further enhances yield,[34] although routine washes are probably not needed if adequate biopsy specimens are taken from a visible lesion. Transbronchoscopic fine needle aspiration of the submucosa and paratracheal and subcarinal nodes has few indications, and is not useful as a routine procedure.[35][36]

Fibreoptic bronchoscopy can be used to diagnose peripheral masses beyond direct vision. It should be a day case procedure whenever possible and pathological results should be available within one week[8]: longer delays are very stressful for patients.

With the advent of fibreoptic bronchoscopy the use of *sputum cytology* has decreased. Indications are now few—for example, an abnormal radiograph and a failed bronchoscopy. Fibreoptic bronchoscopy has a sensitivity and specificity for lung cancer of more than 85%, but the figure for cytology is probably less than 65% even after multiple samples.[37] The processing of sputum, like bronchial washings, is more expensive and difficult than fixed brush smears. Cytological specimens allow accurate diagnosis of squamous cell carcinoma and small cell carcinoma to be made, but typing others, such as poorly differentiated or large cell tumours, is more difficult because of the heterogeneity within them.[38]

81

Thoracic computed tomograms

These are more useful in management than in diagnosis and are pivotal in assessing operability. Although a few centres perform computed tomograms routinely when lung cancer is suspected,[39] this is not routine practice. In view of their cost and the pressure on most scanning units it seems sensible to reserve computed tomograms for particular cases of diagnostic difficulty after plain radiographs and bronchoscopy have been tried. Computed tomograms are particularly good for (a) differentiating pulmonary masses from vessels; (b) showing mediastinal invasion or lymphadenopathy; and (c) demonstrating peripheral pulmonary metastases and pleural anatomy.

Thus computed tomograms may indicate neoplasia when other tests are equivocal. Its major use, overall, is for the difficult hilar shadow with a normal bronchoscopy. The computed tomogram appearances of lymphangitis carcinomatosa are characteristic.[40] This is useful because plain radiographic appearances are often atypical.

Peripheral mass and percutaneous needle biopsy (figure 2)

The dilemma here is whether to observe, investigate, or remove. Even more elaborate algorithms are available.[41] The major point to remember is that evaluation of a peripheral mass involves a simultaneous consideration of the diagnosis and its management and any action taken must depend on the pretest probability of the eventual diagnosis. For example, a peripheral, partly clacified, well circumscribed asymptomatic lesion in a non-smoker of 70 is almost certainly benign and observation with no more investigations can be justified. On the other hand, a slightly irregular, softer density peripheral lesion in a clubbed smoker of the same age is almost certainly a neoplasm and a computed tomogram of the thorax followed, if possible, by excision, is appropriate. Prior knowledge of the cell type will not affect management in either case. By contrast, if a peripheral lesion is unresectable but probably a tumour, then a needle biopsy is almost certainly needed to determine whether chemotherapy (for small cell lung cancer) or radical radiotherapy should be given.

Percutaneous needle biopsy (PCNB) can be done either using fine needle (22 gauge) aspirates for cytology, or larger cutting

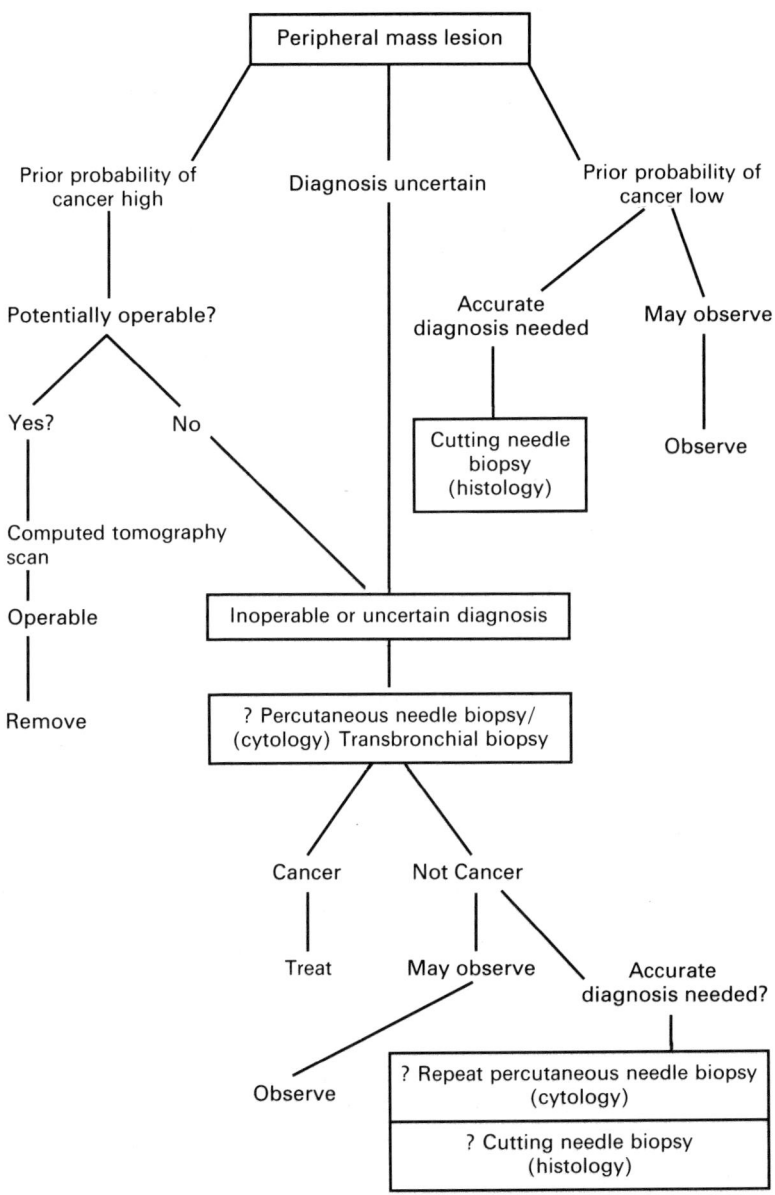

Figure 2   Investigation pathway for peripheral mass lesion.

83

needles, such as Trucut or Rotex, for histology. The specificity for PCNB is nearly 100% for malignancy but its sensitivity is always less, perhaps 80%.[41] Thus a positive result is useful but a negative one does not definitely exclude neoplasia. About 5–10% of passes may fail to obtain diagnostically useful material. The problems of typing tumours using the *cytology* of fine needle aspirates are similar to those of bronchoscopic brushings (see above). A skilled cytopathologist is needed for correct interpretation.

The immediate complication rate is proportional to the needle diameter,[42] the number of passes (one to three), and the depth of the lesion—maximum acceptable depth being 8 cm.[43] Modern imaging is mandatory, either fluoroscopy, computed tomogram, or possibly ultrasound scan if the shadow is adjacent to the pleura. The risk of later problems due to cell dissemination in fine needle tracks is remote.[44 45] This applies not only to lung cancer but also to mesothelioma when fine needles are used.

If the pretest probability of a diagnosis is benign or non-lung cancer malignancy, such as lymphoma, then a cutting needle biopsy is needed and this also has to be considered if a previous fine needle aspirate was negative. In the latter instance the need for a precise pathological diagnosis has to be reviewed.

For cutting needle biopsies most operators use the Trucut needle, or an automatic device. The specificity of sampling is even better than aspiration cytology but the complication rates are higher.[46 47] Experience and good screening are needed. Appropriate pretest checks, such as clotting screens, are mandatory. All cases require a chest radiograph four hours after the test.

Fine needle aspiration can be a day case procedure but cutting needle biopsies usually need an overnight stay in hospital and all cases do so if a pneumothorax is caused. This raises the cost of PCNB from about £200 (equivalent to a fibreoptic bronchoscopy) to about £350.

Some peripheral lesions can be approached by a transbronchial biopsy[48] or transbronchial needle aspiration,[49] at bronchoscopy as part of the screening procedure. This can be combined with bronchial brushing and a segmental saline lavage for cytology. The sensitivity of this approach is only about 50–65%, however, and is particularly low with small lesions.

Finally, the possibility that a coin lesion may be a lone metastasis from a subdiaphragmatic primary, particularly a hypernephroma, must be borne in mind and an upper abdominal ultasound scan before biopsy should be considered in appropriate cases.

Pleural disease (figure 3)

The diagnosis of malignancy derives from needle aspiration of an effusion for protein and cytology, followed by closed pleural biopsy, thoracoscopy, or open pleural biopsy for histology.

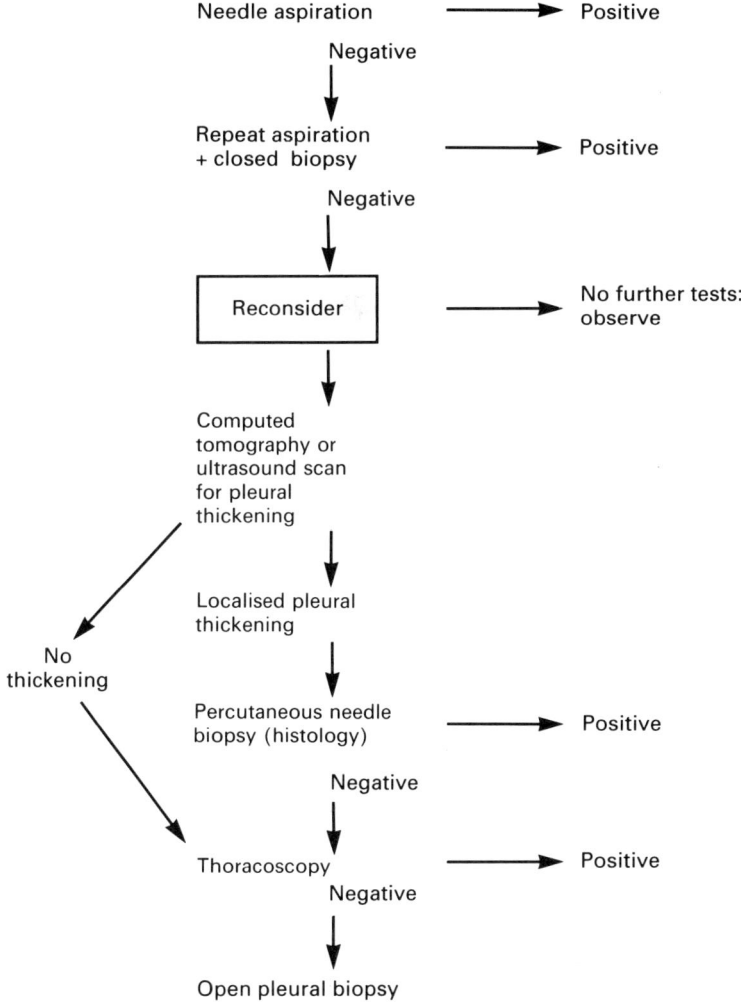

Figure 3   Investigation of pleural disease with high probability of neoplasm.

85

If the local cytology service is rapid and reliable it is probably best to do a simple diagnostic aspiration first. The probability of a transudate (pleural fluid protein of less than 30 g/l) being malignant is very small. The overall sensitivity of a single aspirate is about 60% for malignancy and may rise to 75% if the aspiration is repeated.[50] If the first sample is an exudate with negative cytology and the pre-test probability for cancer is high, however, most physicians would then prefer to perform a repeat aspiration and closed pleural biopsy with multiple samples at the same time.

Figure 3 shows a suggested scheme if no diagnosis is then forthcoming. It is important to remember the possibility of metastatic pleural disease and tuberculosis. Mesothelioma is notoriously difficult to diagnose; reliance may have quite reasonably to be placed on a history of exposure to asbestos and a compatible computed tomogram.

The superior sulcus (Pancoast) tumour is to a certain extent a special case of pleural disease.[51] Sampling with fine needle aspiration under computed tomography is recommended. Management depends crucially on accurate anatomy and this is one of the indications for a magnetic resonance imaging scan.[52 53]

External masses

Lung cancer may occasionally present with a skin mass—either a metastasis or direct spread—or as an enlarged supraclavicular node. PCNB is the diagnostic method of choice. Sensitivity and specificity are very high.[54] Cutting needle biopsy or excision biopsy are needed if either the pretest diagnostic probability is lymphoma, or benign disease, or if the PCNB is negative and the clinical probability of neoplasm remains high.

Mediastinal masses

Again, rarely, lung cancer may present as a mediastinal mass or masses. If this is the working diagnosis then a PCNB is recommended. This can be done under computed tomogram screening or ultrasound scanning if the mass or masses are anterior or posterior.[55] If this test is then negative (no malignant cells) or there is an indication on the smear that the diagnosis may be thymoma or lymphoma, or if review of the working diagnosis shows that it could be either of these two diseases, then a cutting needle biopsy should be done again under scanning control.[55 56] In all other cases open surgical biopsy is required, usually by mediastinotomy or mediastinoscopy.

Summary of diagnostic tests in lung cancer

The usual sequence of diagnostic investigation is shown as an algorithm in figure 3. All patients should be considered for bronchoscopy. A tissue diagnosis should be aimed for unless a considered specialist opinion is that it is not necessary. Most investigations should be done on an outpatient or day case basis. Patients and physicians should expect to have access to rapid accurate cytology, pathology, and radiology services.

The recent large regional surveys in the United Kingdom have shown that a tissue diagnosis is achieved only in about 50–60% of cases. The precise reasons why this figure is not higher are unknown. A proportion of patients are probably considered to have too poor a prognosis because of widespread metastatic disease to justify investigation, and in others attempts to confirm the radiological diagnosis may have failed. There is evidence, however, that the confirmation rate has steadily increased over the past 15 years[7] and there is no reason to suppose that this will not continue.

Management

To discuss the appropriate investigations in the management of lung cancer, we now assume that a diagnosis has been achieved and has appropriate histological support. The first questions to be answered are: is it small cell? (SCLC) and is it (potentially) operable?

Because small cell lung cancer is chemosensitive, it is investigated and managed differently from non-small cell lung cancer (NSCLC) and will be discussed later. The group of non-small cell lung cancer includes all patients with defined histology as well as the large percentage—probably 40% of the total—with no pathological diagnosis,[6] because these patients are managed by physicians as non-small cell lung cancer (figure 4).

Assessment of operability

The initial assessment will have provided evidence that there is not:

1   An absolute general contraindication to surgery—for example, a recent myocardial infarction.
2   Definite bronchoscopic inoperability—for example, carinal tumour.
3   Any feature on the radiograph or at bronchoscopy suggesting

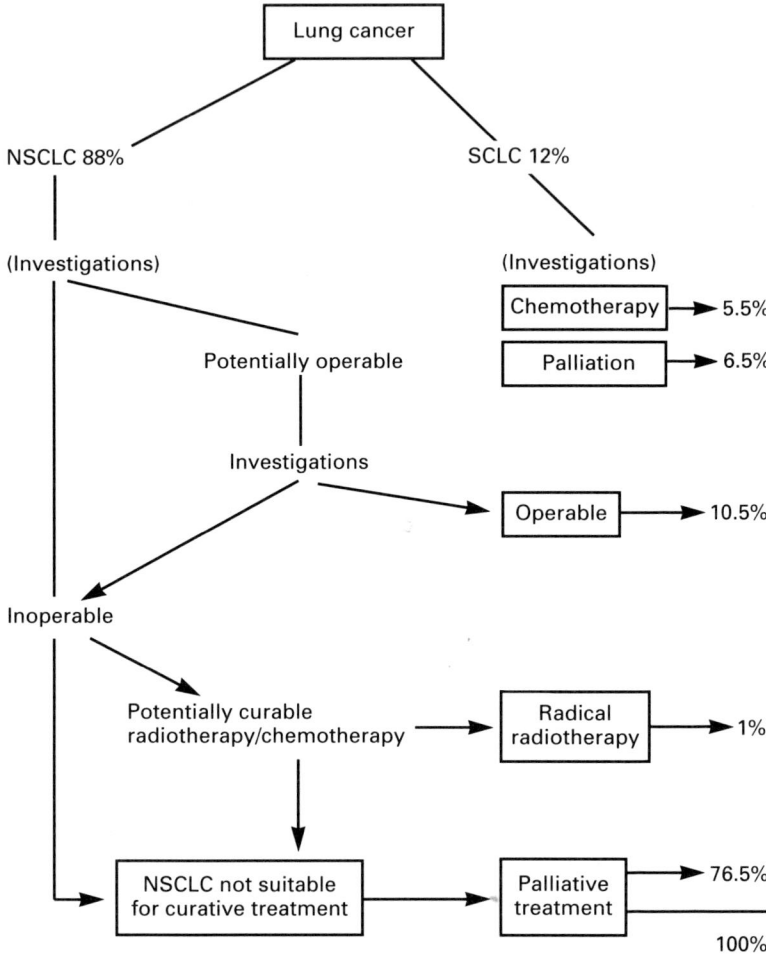

Figure 4 Current picture of lung cancer management in the Yorkshire region (Yorkshire Cancer Registry, 1993). The regional histological confirmation rate is 60%; 20% of these are small cell lung cancer, but this represents only 12% of the total number of cases registered. The 40% without histological confirmation are thus managed effectively as non-small cell lung cancer. 83% of patients with small cell plus non-small cell lung cancer are not suitable for curative treatment after their initial investigations. Operation rates of 10% have been stable for some years.

mediastinal spread; such as a large contralateral nodal mass or carinal widening.

4   Any evidence of metastases.

A detailed discussion of features allowing or disallowing surgery is beyond the scope of this chapter and more details can be found elsewhere.[57] It cannot be emphasised too strongly, however, that specialist advice about operability from a chest physician or a cardiothoracic surgeon is mandatory. The opinion of a cardiothoracic surgeon is the final arbiter and must be obtained in all cases where there is a possibility of a successful curative procedure.

If there are no clearcut contraindications to surgery after the initial assessments all patients should have a computed tomogram of the thorax with contrast (figure 5). Cuts should be taken at the same time across the upper abdomen to include the adrenals and upper liver. Whether physicians without access to computed tomogram scanners should do any other preliminary tests is doubtful. The pickup rate of occult abdominal metastases from upper abdominal ultrasound scans in patients with non-small cell lung cancer of this type is much less than 5%. Ultrasound scanning, however, is widely available, cheap, and has good exclusion value, so it could be done in such cases.

Decision making after computed tomogram scanning has elements of controversy but the following recommendations are made.

1 *The mediastinum is normal*—there is no invasion or nodal enlargement. Even if the hilar nodes are large, the patient should be referred to a cardiothoracic surgeon and thoracotomy recommended with no further tests.

2 *Mediastinal invasion* by the primary lesion precludes surgery.

3 If there is no invasion but *mediastinal nodes are larger than 1 cm* in their short axis diameter[58] the patient should be referred for further investigation.

Comment

Where mediastinal nodes are invaded by tumour (N2) and this is known preoperatively—that is, the patient is stage IIIA—the five year survival is only 5%.[59] If, however, metastases are discovered only when nodes are removed at surgery, previous mediastinal sampling having been negative, the five year survival is about 20–25%.[60 61] In the presence of lung cancer, especially squamous cell, a proportion of enlarged mediastinal nodes are reactive and contain no metastases. A meta analysis in 1989 of 42 studies, comparing computed tomogram scan results with node histology, showed that

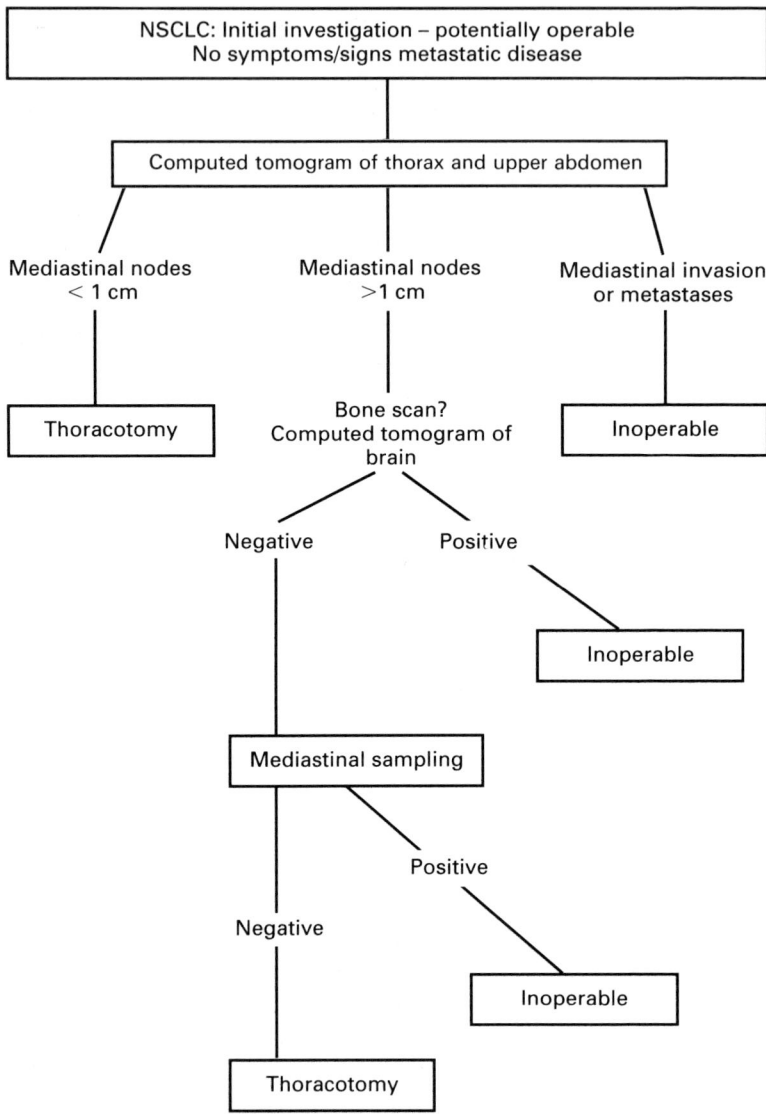

Figure 5   Scanning and mediastinal sampling in potentially operable patients with NSCLC.

if a cut off value of greater than 1 cm in diameter for the short axis was used to define an abnormal node, the sensitivity of computed tomography scanning was 79% and its specificity 86%.[62] Thus, overall, computed tomography scanning has *at least* a 20% false positive and false negative rate, and more recent studies with detailed node mapping have indicated higher figures than this.[63 64] Even though large nodes are more likely to be malignant, careful studies have shown that a proportion of even these are benign. In McLeod's study[63] 13% (43) of 336 nodes of less than 1 cm diameter contained metastases, 25% (14) of 57 1·0–1·9 cm, and 67% (15) of 21 greater than 2 cm in diameter. For all nodes greater than 1 cm, only 36% had metastases. It is therefore clear that node size alone on a computed tomogram scan should not determine inoperability. Mediastinal sampling is recommended for all these cases,[65] although it is not universal practice at present in the United Kingdom,[66] and so many futile thoracotomies are still carried out—16% of all listed in the United Kingdom thoracic surgical register of 1988.

The cost and outcomes of different managements can be compared. Assuming that 60 out of 100 patients with enlarged nodes on computed tomograms have no metastases and can have curative resections, then a policy of mediastinal sampling in all cases would lead to the 100 patients having this done and 60 having subsequent surgery. Without mediastinal sampling, 100 thoracotomies would be done, 40 of which would be futile. Thus 100 mediastinoscopies costing, say, £135 000 save 40 thoracotomies costing about £320 000, a financial saving of 65%, together with a large reduction in patient morbidity.

Scanning for metastases preoperatively

It is pointless to recommend a thoracotomy if the patient already has distant metastases. Clearly any suggestive symptoms or abnormal biochemistry would demand appropriate investigation. A more difficult question is: What, if any, preoperative scans should be done in asymptomatic patients? There is now good evidence that, not surprisingly, patients with N2 disease have a greater probability of such metastases than patients with N0 or N1 disease. Thus Grant et al[68] showed that only three out of 77 (4%) of patients with a normal mediastinum preoperatively on a computed tomogram scan had occult metastases found in concurrent computed tomogram scans of the brain and abdomen; 12 of 37 (32%) with an abnormal mediastinum did so.

There have been only five other similar studies so far.[69-73] The number of patients found to have metastases, although operable on the basis of a previous computed tomogram of the thorax, were as follows:

for the brain (computed tomogram) five of 392 (1·2%)[68 69 72 73];
for liver and adrenals combined (computed tomogram scan) eight of 354 (2%)[68 69 70 72];
for bone (isotope scan, clinical follow up) 16 of 343 (4·6%).[69 70-72]

Michel et al[71] showed that *no* bone metastases were detected in a very carefully followed up series of patients who initially had *no* known biochemical abnormality, or *any* symptoms suggestive of bone metastases.

Most computed tomogram units, when asked for a computed tomogram scan of the thorax in this context, would now scan the upper abdomen with contrast at the same time. This halves the cost of investigating the abdomen. Thus the management problem reduces to whether routine computed tomogram brain and isotope bone scans are justified by the low pickup rate in these patients.

At present there are insufficient data for a completely clear answer, and in any case the decision may depend on an unquantifiable attitude towards the cost:benefit ratios. In terms of the financial costs alone, for example, the above data indicate that more than 25 bone scans and computed tomogram brain scans (estimated cost £3000) would be needed, on average, in these patients to detect one unexpected metastasis and prevent one thoracotomy (estimated cost £8000 to GP fund holders).

In the author's view the practical conclusion should be that patients with a normal mediastinum do not need these scans as it is likely that more than 95% of them will be normal. Patients with enlarged mediastinal nodes (N2 or stage III disease) on computed tomography should be investigated.

It seems sensible to recommend for these patients:

(1) a bone scan if there are any suggestive symptoms or biochemical abnormalities;
(2) further abdominal investigations if the computed tomogram scan of the chest has not included the upper abdomen and this was normal; and
(3) a computed tomography brain scan.

These scans should, in the author's opinion, probably precede mediastinal sampling (figure 5). Mediastinal sampling could, in theory, be considered first if some nodes are greater than 2 cm in diameter as the chance of these being metastatic is over 60%; the chance of occult metastases being discovered is much less. Mediastinal sampling, however, costs about £1300, and a bone scan and a computed tomography brain scan together cost about £200, with no requirement for inpatient stay and no operative risk.

Fitness for surgery

At present an electrocardiogram, spirometry, and an informal exercise test, such as stair climbing, are the norm. Few centres routinely perform more elaborate tests, but these are necessary: (1) if there is evidence of angina; (2) the FEV1 is less than 1·2 litres or less than 30% predicted; or the FEV1/FVC is less than 60% predicted[74 75]; (3) exercise tolerance seems poor and the patient is regarded as borderline for surgery.

Lobectomy reduces the FEV1 and FVC by about 10—15% predicted and pneumonectomy by 20–30% predicted. The risks of postoperative morbidity and disability are high if the postoperative FEV1 is likely to be less than 0·8 litres to 1·0 litres or less than 30% predicted.[76] Postoperative lung function and exercise tolerance can be predicted accurately from a combination of spirometry and quantitative perfusion lung scans.[77 78] Although a VO_2 max of less than 50 ml/kg/minute measured in a formal exercise test is associated with greater perioperative risk and postoperative morbidity,[79] simpler tests are probably as accurate.[78] The transfer factor may be helpful because the postoperative complication rate is higher if there is less than 40% predicted.[76] As well as these tests, a measure of 6 minute walking distance[80] and a short period of intensive exercise training and bronchodilation are recommended in borderline cases before a decision not to operate is made. In practice, the number of patients successfully undergoing resection and yet who have disabling breathlessness appears to be small.

Management of inoperable patients potentially suitable for other treatment

The small proportion of patients with stage I or stage II disease who for general medical, technical, or psychological reasons do not come to surgery may be cured by radical radiotherapy. Investigation of these patients should, logically, be along the same lines as surgical candidates if the goal of treatment is cure.

Patients with more advanced local disease can be considered for "disease-modifying" rather than palliative radiotherapy and need to have their local disease assessed by thoracic computed tomogram scans. As the incidence of occult metastases is likely to be over 10%, it seems sensible to consider organ scanning along the lines above if an extended course of radiotherapy is being considered. Mediastinal sampling is not required.

In the same way, adequate staging of patients before planned chemotherapy is recommended. Because the benefit of chemotherapy for non-small cell lung cancer is controversial, patients should normally be treated with trial protocols and investigated accordingly.[81]

Management of patients not able to have treatment to improve their prognosis

Figure 1 shows that more than 80% of patients currently presenting with lung cancer fall into this category. This is about 28 000 a year in the United Kingdom or 150 per health district—nine times as many as can be considered for curative treatment.

Furthermore, lung cancer is increasingly a disease which occurs in the over 70s. Twenty per cent of all cases recorded by the Yorkshire Cancer Registry in 1975–6 were over 75, and this increased to 31% in 1988–9.[7] The typical patient will now be living alone or with a less than fit spouse. The continuing care of patients cannot be accomplished under these circumstances without some investigation and knowledge of these conditions. Sensible use of Macmillan nurses and medical social workers may be far more important to the patient later on in the disease than more minor physical symptoms, some of which these elderly smokers may have been used to for many years.

The published data on the investigation of lung cancer for management are dominated by the assessment of operability. Investigation of inoperable patients has received far less attention. Nevertheless, this is a much larger problem and deserves the same careful approach. Correct management again depends on a logical assessment of the disease. This needs:

(1)   separate estimates of symptoms due to the primary lesion and metastases, and which of these can be relieved by antitumour treatment;
(2)   an estimate of which of these symptoms and any paraneoplastic symptoms can be relieved by other palliative measures;
(3)   an estimate of the patient's psychological state and social support;
(4)   an estimate of the prognosis.

Investigations are only justified if treatment follows and this in turn can be expected to produce a worth while duration of benefit. Estimating prognosis is difficult. A recent study of the accuracy of five physicians and radiotherapists managing 300 patients showed that they tended to be optimistic. Forty nine (16%) more patients were predicted to survive more than three months and 36 (13%) more than six months than actually did so.[82] Conversely, however, the specificity of physicians' opinions on accuracy when they *predicted* survival to be less than three months was 96%.

Chest symptoms

Patients with respiratory symptoms need sufficient tests to determine whether their symptoms are due to lung cancer, whether palliative treatment of this may help, and secondly to establish whether there are any alternative diagnoses. There are numerous possibilities, but most patients with troublesome symptoms of this type need a combination of a chest radiograph and a lateral, bronchoscopy, and spirometry. These tests should determine whether palliative external beam radiotherapy, local endobronchial treatment,[83] or bronchodilator treatment[84] will help. Symptoms due to mediastinal spread, such as dysphagia, superior venal caval obstruction, hoarseness or pain may need additional tests—for example, a barium swallow, endoscopy, a bone scan or occasionally a thoracic computed tomogram. Pleural disease requires plain radiographs with ultrasound scanning or occasionally computed tomography for more difficult cases. Cardiac symptoms such as dysrhythmias or a suspicion of breathlessness due to pericardial effusion would probably best be investigated by echocardiography which may show a surprisingly high proportion of unsuspected pericardial spread in patients with mediastinal disease.[85]

Metastatic disease

For metastatic disease the first rule of investigation is to do no special tests without a *scrupulous* history and examination, together with plain radiology. If this is not done patients will have scans of no value. Thereafter which special tests to do is usually quite clear. Skin metastases rarely need PCNB. For bone symptoms, an isotope scan is recommended in addition to plain radiographs for localisation when palliative radiotherapy or other local intervention is being considered. Brain scans are required if the diagnosis is in doubt, and will allow radiotherapy to be planned and a more accurate prognosis given. There remain a number of patients who have more diffuse unexplained central nervous system symptoms such as confusion or inattention, and a brain scan in these cases may help too.

As access to computed tomography scanners is improving, the need for the less reliable isotope brain scan is diminishing, although these can be used on occasion to demonstrate large metastases.

Upper abdominal ultrasound scanning is the best test to investigate a clinical suspicion of symptomatic abdominal metastases—notably, in the liver, nodes, or retroperitoneal organs.

Paraneoplastic syndromes

Every doctor caring for patients with lung cancer must know that some of these syndromes are common and that they can on occasion explain otherwise "inexplicable" physical symptoms. A combination of meticulous history and examination together with blood tests will diagnose most of them (table I).

Psychological symptoms

Psychological symptoms may be difficult to disentangle from physical debility. The hospital anxiety and depression scale[86] is a well validated and useful instrument which is easy to apply.

Time lapse between referral and start of treatment

There are few data on the usual interval between referral from the general practitioner and treatment for lung cancer. Figures from the Yorkshire Cancer Registry 1988–91 showed that the median delay for the 40% of patients throughout the region who had definitive anti-cancer treatment—surgery, radiotherapy, or chemotherapy—was 12 days between referral and first hospital

TABLE I   Presentations due to paraneoplastic syndromes

Symptoms and signs	Abnormality
Common:	
Fatigue, anorexia, weight loss	Abnormal cellular metabolism due to? tumour necrosis factor
Fatigue	Anaemia of chronic disease
Weakness, sickness, thirst	Hypercalcaemia: parathyroid hormone peptide
Fatigue, weakness	Hyponatraemia (syndrome of inappropriate secretion of antidiuretic hormone)
Rare:	
Muscle weakness and skin rash	Dermatomyositis
Myasthenia-like weakness	Eaton Lambert syndrome
Paraesthesiae/sensory loss	Peripheral neuropathy
Limb pains and tenderness	HPOA
Skin rash	Acanthosis nigricans
Visual failure	Retinal damage: autoantibodies
Repeated deep venous thromboses	Thrombophlebitis migrans
Weakness	Hypokalaemic alkalosis (adreno-corticotrophic hormone-like peptide)
Proteinuria, oedema, renal failure	Nephrotic syndrome
Breathlessness, heart murmur	Marantic endocarditis
Episodic faintness	Spontaneous hypoglycaemia

HPOA: Hypertrophic pulmonary osteoarthropathy.

visit (interquartile range 6–20) and 22 days between this hospital visit and the start of treatment (11 to 40 days).

Small cell lung cancer

This diagnosis will have been made as part of the initial assessment and can only be based on histology or cytology. The diagnosis of small cell lung cancer using pleural fluid cytology alone is somewhat unreliable but other cytological specimens are accurate. In contrast to non-small cell lung cancer, bone marrow examination is a useful additional test to consider in cases of difficulty.

Prognosis and staging

Prognostic factors for small cell lung cancer have been widely researched and the most powerful pretreatment factors are performance status, disease extent, and biochemical measurements of

97

sodium, alkaline phosphatase, lactate dehydrogenase or abumin, and aspartate aminotransferase.[87] The concept of performance status or activity score was introduced by Karnofsky.[88] It is essentially a clinical measure of how a disease affects an individual's overall function (table II). A similar index has been developed by the World Health Organisation.[89]

The tumour, nodes, metastases (TNM) classification which correlates strongly with prognosis in non-small cell lung cancer is not applicable in small cell lung cancer because of the very high rate of distant metastases at presentation, sometimes coming from small primaries with no adjacent lymphadenopathy. Patients are therefore divided generally into two groups: those with "limited" disease confined to the ipsilateral thorax and ipsilateral supraclavicular fossa, including a pleural effusion; and "extensive disease" — all other patients. At the time of presentation more than 70% of patients have extensive disease. It has to be remembered, however,

TABLE II Comparison of indices of performance status

Karnofsky index		Zubrod-ECOG-WHO scale	
Status	*Score*	*Score*	*Status*
Normal; no complaints	100	0	Normal activity
Able to carry on normal activities	90	1	Symptoms, but nearly ambulatory
Minor signs or symptoms of disease			
Normal activity with effort	80		
Cares for self; unable to carry on normal activity or to do active work	70	2	Some time in bed, but needs to be in bed less than 50% of normal daytime
Requires occasional assistance, but able to care for most needs	60		
Requires considerable assistance and frequent medical care	50	3	Needs to be in bed more than 50% of normal daytime
Disabled; requires special care and assistance	40		
Severely disabled; hospitalisation indicated, though death not imminent	30	4	Unable to get out of bed
Very sick; hospitalisation necessary; active supportive treatment necessary	20		
Moribund	10		
Dead	0		

that the more scanning that is done the more patients will move from the limited to the extensive category, with the probability of an apparent increase in survival of both groups. Therefore, in a sense the current method of staging small cell lung cancer is arbitrary, although prognostic scores which correlate with survival are used as the basis for allocating patients to different treatment policies. In this context routine organ scanning in this disease adds little, and the essential management information is that listed above.[89-93] Moreover, multiple scanning can delay treatment for several weeks, during which some patients may become unfit for active intervention, given the rapid growth of small cell lung cancer.

Because of the high incidence of metastases, the physician has to have a high index of suspicion with regard to minor abnormalities in the initial assessment. For example, abnormal liver function tests and *any* neurological symptoms have to be assumed to be due to neoplastic disease until there is evidence to the contrary.

The median survival of untreated small cell lung cancer is less than three months. This single figure disguises a wide variation, however, ranging from the patient with a better prognosis and good performance status and limited disease to the bed-fast or restricted patient with extensive metastases. All patients should be considered for chemotherapy, however, preferably within a setting of a clinical trial. The reason for this is that optimal strategies for different prognostic groups have not been defined. Recent research has shown that as few as three courses of chemotherapy may be appropriate for some of the patients with poorer prognosis in that they can be treated with simple combinations of drugs. Furthermore, modern anti-emetic treatments have reduced the side effects of treatment. At the other end of the spectrum, in contrast, up to six courses of multiple drug treatment, combined with radiotherapy, are now standard. Most patients will not require multiple scans or even computed tomography of the thorax, and fitness for chemotherapy is defined by an assessment of the performance status, and the demonstration that the patient does not have severe hepatic, renal, or bone marrow dysfunction.

Patients with these abnormalities and those who are severely symptomatic or who are moribund with the prognosis of only a few weeks should not be considered for multiple drug chemotherapy, and palliative treatment should be regarded as more appropriate.

Symptomatic metastases require appropriate radiographs and occasionally scans as rapid palliation results from short courses of radiotherapy.

Patients up to 75 years of age have been shown to benefit from multiple drug chemotherapy. The fitness of people older than this is questionable and again expert oncological advice is necessary. Such patients should not be denied this advice on the basis of age alone.

Conclusion

Good management of patients with lung cancer is difficult and time consuming. Expert advice is needed in most cases from an interested chest physician, cardiothoracic surgeon, medical oncologist or radiotherapist, or members of a palliative care team. For non-specialists, probably the best investigation is, in fact, a consultation note.

I thank Mrs Lesley Rider of the Yorkshire Cancer Registry for permission to quote data from the reports. Thanks are due to Dr P J Robinson, director, Department of Radiology, St James's University Hospital, for providing estimates of investigation costs; to Mrs Kim Gaye, financial services director, United Leeds Teaching Hospital NHS Trust, for providing cost estimates for inpatient procedures; and to Mrs Elaine A Power for her dedicated secretarial assistance.

1 Bernhard J, Ganz PA. Psychosocial issues in lung cancer patients (2). *Chest* 1991;**99**:480–5.

2 Medical Research Council. Inoperable non small cell lung cancer. Medical Research Council randomised trial of palliative radiotherapy with 2 fractions or 10 fractions. *Br J Cancer* 1991;**63**:265–70.

3 Medical Research Council Lung Cancer Working Party. Respective randomised trial of 3 or 6 courses of etoposide, cyclophosphamide, methotrexate and vincristine and of 6 courses of etoposide and ifosfamide in small cell lung cancer (SCLC). *Lung Cancer* 1991;1(Suppl 103):378A.

4 Hetzel MR, Smith SGT. Endoscopic palliation of tracheobronchial malignancies. *Thorax* 1991;**46**:325–33.

5 Goldman JM, Bulman AS, Rathmell AJ, Carey BM, Muers MF, Joslin CAF. Physiological effect of endobronchial radiotherapy in patients with major airway occlusion by carcinoma. *Thorax* 1993;**48**:110–14.

6 Connolly CK, Jones WG, Thorogood J, Head C, Muers MF. Investigation, treatment and prognosis of bronchial carcinoma in the Yorkshire Region of England. 1976–1983. *Br J Cancer* 1990;**61**:579–83.

7 *Cancer in Yorkshire: Cancert Registry Report Special Series 1. Lung Cancer.* Leeds: Yorkshire Regional Cancer Organisation, 1993.

8 Muers MF, Chappell AG, Farebrother M, Farrow SC, Harrison BDW, Lazlo G. Facilities for the diagnosis of respiratory disease in the UK. *J Roy Coll Phys* 1988;**22**:180–4.

9 Fletcher F, Johnston RN, Stradling P. The normal chest radiograph in bronchial carcinoma. *Br Med J* 1976;**2**:403.

10 Austin JHM, Romney BM, Goldsmith LS. Missed bronchogenic carcinoma: radiographic findings in 27 patients with a potentially resectable lesion evident in retrospect. *Radiology* 1992;**182**:115–22.

11 Cooper EH, Splinter TAW, Brown DA, Muers MF, Peake MD, Pearson SB. Evaluation of a radioimmunoassay for neuron specific enolase in small cell lung cancer. *Br J Cancer* 1985;**52**:333–8.
12 Gomm SA, Keevil BG, Thatcher N, Hasleton P, Swindell RS. Value of tumour markers in lung cancer. *Br J Cancer* 1988;**58**:797–804.
13 Jorgensen LGM, Hansen HH, Cooper EH. Neuron specific enolase, carcinoembryonic antigen and lactic dehydrogenase as indicators of disease activity in small cell lung cancer. *Eur J Cancer Clin Oncol* 1989;**25**:123–8.
14 Miyake M, Taki T, Hitomi S, Hakomori S-I. Correlation of expression of H/Le^y/Le^b antigens with survival in patients with carcinoma of the lung. *N Engl J Med* 1992;**327**:12–18.
15 Lee JS, Hong WK. Prognostic factors in lung cancer. *N Engl J Med* 1992;**327**:47–8.
16 Gislason T, Nou E. Sedimentation rate, leucocytes, platelet count, and haemoglobin in bronchial carcinoma: an epidemiological study. *Eur J Respir Dis* 1985;**66**:141–6.
17 Marshall RJ, Curzon PDG, Pearson SB, Cooper EH, Muers MF, Peake MD. Prognosis in squamous cell lung cancer: the contribution of plasma proteins. *Tumor Diagnost Ther* 1985;**6**:195–8.
18 Hanson P, Collins J. Bronchoscopy and lavage. In Brewis RAL, Gibson GJ, Geddes DM, eds. *Respiratory medicine*. London: Ballière Tindall, 1990:316–29.
19 Muers MF. Bronchoscopy and tissue biopsy. In Weatherall DJ, Ledingham JGG, Warrell DA, eds. *Oxford textbook of medicine*. 2nd Edn. Oxford: OUP, 1987:15.7–15.10.
20 Fulkerson WJ. Current concepts: Fiberoptic bronchoscopy. *N Engl J Med* 1982;**311**:511–15.
21 Reed AP. Preparation of the patient for awake flexible fiberoptic bronchoscopy. *Chest* 1992;**101**:244–53.
22 Webb AR, Doherty JF, Chester MR, *et al.* Sedation for fibreoptic bronchoscopy: comparison of alfentanyl with papaveretum and diazepam. *Respir Med* 1989;**83**:213–17.
23 Goreszfeniuk T, Nicholas IH, Marchant P, *et al.* Premedication for fibreoptic bronchoscopy: Fentenyl, diazepam and atropine compared with papaveretum and hyoscine. *Br Med J* 1980;**281**:486.
24 Pearce SJ. Fibreoptic bronchoschopy: Is sedation really necessary? *Br Med J* 1986;**221**:779–80.
25 Dubrawsky C, Awer J, Jenkins DE. The effect of bronchofiberscopic examination on oxygenation status. *Chest* 1975;**67**:137–40.
26 Teale C, Gomes PJ, Muers MF, Pearson SB. Local anaesthetic for fibreoptic bronchoscopy: comparison between intra tracheal cocaine and lignocaine. *Respir Med* 1990;**84**:407–9.
27 Middleton RM, Shah A, Kirkpatrick MB. Topical nasal anaesthesia for fiberoptic bronchoscopy. *Chest* 1991;**99**:1093–6.
28 Simpson FG, Arnold AG, Purvis A, Belfield PW, Muers MF, Cooke NJ. Postal survey of bronchoscopic practice by physicians in the United Kingdom. *Thorax* 1986;**41**:311–17.
29 Prakash UBS, Offord KP, Stubbs SE. Bronchoscopy in North America: the ACCP survey. *Chest* 1991;**100**:1668–75.
30 Knox AJ, Mascie-Taylor BH, Page RL. Fibreoptic bronchoscopy in the elderly: 4 years experience. *Br J Dis Chest* 1988;**82**:290–3.
31 Macfarlane JT, Storr A, Ward MJ, Roderick-Smith WH. Safety, usefulness and acceptability of fibreoptic bronchoscopy in the elderly. *Age Ageing* 1981;**10**:172–31.
32 Gellert AR, Rudd RM, Sinha G, Geddes DM. Fibreoptic bronchoscopy: effect of multiple biopsies on diagnostic yield in bronchial carcinoma. *Thorax* 1982;**37**:684–7.
33 Muers MF, Boddington MM, Cole M, Murphy D, Spriggs AI. Cytological sampling at fibreoptic bronchoscopy: a comparison of catheter aspirates and brush biopsies. *Thorax* 1982;**37**:457–61.
34 Mak VHF, Johnston IDA, Hetzel MR, Grubb C. Value of washings and brushings at fibreoptic bronchoscopy in diagnosis of lung cancer. *Thorax* 1990;**45**:373–6.
35 Blaney AD, Carling M, Green M. Transbronchial aspiration of subcarinal lymph nodes. *Br J Dis Chest* 1988;**82**:149–54.
36 Harrow EM, Oldenburg FA, Jr, Lingenfelter MS, Marshall-Smith A. Transbronchial needle aspiration in clinical practice. A five year experience. *Chest* 1989;**16**:1268–72.
37 Johnston WW, Bossen EH. Ten years of respiratory cytopathology at Duke University Medical Center. 1. The cytopathologic diagnosis of lung cancer during the years 1970–1974 noting the significance of specimen number and type. *Acta Cytol* 1981;**25**:103–7.

38 DiBonito L, Colautti I, Patriavca S, Falconieri C, Barbazza R, Vielh P. Cytological typing of primary lung cancer: study of 100 cases with autopsy confirmation. *Diagnost Cytopathol* 1991;**7**:7–10.

39 Gommersall LN, Duncan KA, Weir J, Cairns J, Jeffrey RR. An evaluation of extrathoracic metastatic disease in potentially resectable non small cell bronchogenic carcinoma: implications for staging. *Thorax* 1993;**48**:441.

40 Stein MG, Mayo J, Muller N. Pulmonary lymphangitic spread of carcinoma: appearance on CT scans. *Radiology* 1987;**162**:137–40.

41 Caskey CI. Zerhooni EA. The solitary pulmonary nodule. *Semin Roentgenol* 1990;**25**:85–95.

42 Young CP, Young I, Cowan DF, Blei R. The reliability of fine-needle aspiration biopsy in the diagnosis of deep lesions of the lung and mediastinum: experience with 250 cases using a modified technique. *Diagnost Ctyopathol* 1987;**3**:1–7.

43 Poe RH, Kallay MC, Wicks CM, Odoroff CL. Predicting the risk of pneumothorax in needle biopsy of the lung. *Chest* 1984;**85**:232–5.

44 Mooloo Z, Finley RJ, Lefcoe MS, Turner-Smith L, Craig ID. Possible spread of bronchogenic carcinoma to the chest wall after a transthoracic fine needle aspiration biopsy: a case report. *Acta Cytol* 1985;**29**:167–9.

45 Voravud N, Shin DM, Dekmezian RH, Dimery I, Lee JS, Jong WK. Implantation metastasis of carcinoma after percutaneous fine-needle aspiration biopsy. *Chest* 1992;**102**:313–4.

46 McEvoy RD, Begley MD, Antic R. Percutaneous biopsy of intrapulmonary mass lesions. *Cancer* 1983;**51**:2321–6.

47 Harrison BDW, Thorpe RS, Kitchener PG, McCann BG, Pillinge JR. Percutaneous Trucut biopsy in the diagnosis of localised pulmonary lesions. *Thorax* 1984;**39**:493–9.

48 Wallace JM, Deutsch AL. Flexible fiberoptic bronchoscopy and percutaneous needle aspiration for evaluation of the solitary pulmonary nodule. *Chest* 1982;**81**:665–71.

49 Harrow E, Halber M, Hardy T, Halteman W. Bronchoscopic and roentgenographic correlates of a positive transbronchial needle aspiration in the staging of lung cancer. *Chest* 1991;**100**:1592–6.

50 Salyer WA, Eggleston JC, Erozan YS. Efficacy of pleural needle biopsy and pleural fluid cytopathology in the diagnosis of malignant neoplasm involving the pleura. *Chest* 1975;**67**:536–9.

51 O'Connell RS, McCloud TL, Wilkins EW. Superior sulcus tumor. Radiographic diagnosis and workup. *Am J Roentgenol* 1983;**140**:25–30.

52 Rapoport S, Blair DN, McCarthy SM. Brachial plexus: correlation of MR imaging with CT and pathologic findings. *Radiology* 1988;**167**:161–5.

53 Gefter W. Magnetic resonance imaging in the evaluation of lung cancer. *Semin Roentgenol* 1990;**25**:73–84.

54 Frable WJ. *Thin needle aspiration biopsy*. Philadelphia: WB Saunders, 1983.

55 Saito T, Kobayashi H, Sugama Y, Tamaki S, Kawai T, Kitamura S. Ultrasonically guided needle biopsy in the diagnosis of mediastinal masses. *Am Rev Respir Dis* 1988;**138**:679–84.

56 Sawhney S, Jain R, Berry M. Trucut biopsy of mediastinal masses guided by real-time sonography. *Clin Radiol* 1991;**41**:16–19.

57 Ginsberg RJ, Goldberg M, Waters PF. Surgery for non-small lung cancer. In: Roth JA, Ruckdeschel JC, Weisenburger TH. *Thoracic oncology*. Philadelphia: WB Saunders, 1989: 177–99.

58 Ingram CE, Belliam, Lewars MD, *et al*. Normal lymph node size in the mediastinum: A retrospective study in two patient groups. *Clin Radiol* 1989;**40**:35–9.

59 Gibbons JRP. The value of mediastinoscopy in assessing operability in carcinoma of the lung. *Br J Dis Chest* 1972;**66**:162–6.

60 Sawamura K, Mori T, Hashimoto S, *et al*. Results of surgical treatment of N2 disease. *Lung Cancer* 1986;**2**:96–101.

61 Martini N, Flehinger B, Zaman M, Beattie EJ Jr, *et al*. Prospective study of 445 lung carcinomas with mediastinal lymph node metastases. *J Thorac Cardiovasc Surg* 1980;**80**:390–7.

62 Dales RE, Stark R, Sanicaranarayanan R. Computed tomography to stage lung cancer: approaching a controversy using meta analysis. *Am Rev Respir Dis* 1990;**141**:1096–101.

63 McLeod TC, Bourgouin PM, Greenberg RW, *et al*. Bronchogenic carcinoma: analysis of staging in the mediastinum with CT by correlative lymph node mapping and sampling. *Radiol* 1992;**182**:319–23.

64 Whittlesey D. Prospective computed tomographic scanning in the staging of bronchogenic cancer. *J Thorac Cardiovasc Surg* 1988;**95**:876–82.
65 Goldstraw P. The practice of cardiothoracic surgeons in the pre-operative staging of lung cancer. *Thorax* 1992;**47**:1–2.
66 Tsang GMK, Watson DCT. The practice of cardiothoracic surgeons in the perioperative staging of non small-cell lung cancer. *Thorax* 1992;**47**:3–5.
67 Sanderson H, Mountney L, Harris J. *Purchasing for cancer of the lung.* Wessex Cancer Intelligence Unit, 1992.
68 Grant D, Edwards D, Goldstraw P. Computed tomography of the brain, chest and abdomen in the pre-operative assessment of non-small cell lung cancer. *Thorax* 1988;**43**:883–6.
69 Doyle PT, Weir J, Robertson EM, Foote AV, Cockburn JS. Role of computed tomography in assessing "operability" of bronchial carcinoma. *Br Med J* 1986;**292**:231–3.
70 Heavey LR, Glazer GM, Gross BH, Francis IR, Orringer MB. The role of CT in staging radiographic T₁ NoMo lung cancer. *Am J Radiol* 1986;**146**:285–90.
71 Michel F, Soler F, Soler M, Imhof E, Perruchoud AP. Initial staging of non-small cell lung cancer: Value of routine radioisotope bone scanning. *Thorax* 1991;**46**:469–73.
72 Salvatherra A, Baabionde C, Llamas C, Cruz F, Lopez-Pugol J. Extrathoracic staging of bronchogenic carcinoma. *Chest* 1990;**97**:1052–8.
73 Salbeck R, Grau HC, Artmann H. Cerebral tumour staging in patients with bronchial carcinoma by computed tomography. *Cancer* 1999;**66**:2007–1.
74 Lockwood P. Lung function test results and the risk of post thoracotomy complications. *Respiration* 1973;**30**:529–42.
75 Miller JI, Grossman GD, Hatcher CR. Pulmonary function test: criteria for operability and pulmonary resection. *Surg Gynaecol Obstet* 1981;**153**:893–5.
76 Gass GD, Olsen GN. Pre-operative pulmonary function testing to predict post operative morbidity and mortality. *Chest* 1986;**89**:127–35.
77 Wernly JA, Demeester TR, Kirchner PT, *et al.* Clinical value of quantitative ventilation—perfusion lung scans in the surgical management of bronchogenic carcinoma. *J Thorac Cardiovasc Surg* 1980;**80**:533–43.
78 Corris PA, Ellis DA, Hawkins T, Gibson GJ. Use of radionuclide scanning in the preoperative estimation of pulmonary function after resection. *Thorax* 1987;**42**:285–91.
79 Smith TP, Kinasewitz GT, Tucker WY, Spillers WP, George RS. Exercise capacity as a predictor of post-thoracotomy morbidity. *Am Rev Respir Dis* 1984;**129**:730–4.
80 Knox AJ, Morrison JFJ, Muers MF. Reproducibility of walking test results in chronic obstructive airways disease. *Thorax* 1988;**43**:388–92.
81 Cullen MH, Joshi R, Chetiyawardana AD, Woodroffe CM. Mitomycin, Ifosamide and Cisplatin in non-small cell lung cancer: treatment good enough to compare. *Br J Cancer* 1988;**58**:359–61.
82 Muers MF. Survival in non-small cell lung cancer [NSCLC]: physicians' opinion compared with prognostic factors. *Thorax* 1990;**45**:804.
83 Hetzel MR, Smith CGT. Endoscopic palliation of tracheobronchial malignancies. *Thorax* 1991;**46**:325–33.
84 Congleton J, Muers MF. Bronchial carcinoma, airflow obstruction and breathlessness. *Thorax* 1992;**47**:862.
85 Corris PA, Kertes PJ, Jennings K, Morritt GN, Neville E, Gibson GJ. Detection of occult cardiac invasion by two dimensional echocardiography in patients with bronchial carcinoma. *Thorax* 1986;**46**:138–41.
86 Zigmond AS, Snaith RP. The hospital anxiety and depression scale. *Acta Psychiatr Scand* 1983;**67**:361–70.
87 Rawson NSB, Peto J. An overview of prognostic factors in small cell lung cancer. A report from the subcommittee for the management of lung cancer, of the United Kingdom coordinated committee of cancer research. *Br J Cancer* 1990;**61**:597–604.
88 Karnofsky DA, Burchenal JH. The clinical evaluation of chemotherapeutic agents in cancer [1949]. In: MacLeod CM, ed. *Evaluation of chemotherapeutic agents.* New York: Columbia Press.
89 WHO. *Handbook for reporting results of cancer treatment. WHO offset publication No 48.* Geneva: WHO, 1979.
90 Osterlind K, Andersen PK. Prognostic factors in small-cell cancer: multivariate model based on 778 patients treated with chemotherapy with or without irradiation. *Cancer Res* 1986;**46**:4189–94.

91 Vincent MD, Ashley SE, Smith RE. Prognostic factors in small cell lung cancer: A simple prognostic index is better than conventional staging. *Eur J Cancer* 1987;**23**:1589–99.

92 Cerny T, Blair V, Anderson H, *et al*. Pre-treatment prognostic factors and scoring system in 407 small cell lung cancer patients. *Int J Cancer* 1987;**39**:146–9.

93 Souhami RL, Bradbury I, Geddes DM, Spiro SG, Harper PG, Tobias JS. Prognostic significance of laboratory parameters measured at diagnosis. *Cancer Res* 1985;**45**:2878–82.

7 Recent clinical trials in advanced lung cancer

DAVID J GIRLING, NICHOLAS W THATCHER

A survey on the impact of clinical trials on the treatment of lung cancer in the United Kingdom[1] showed that in 1991 only 40% of newly diagnosed patients were referred to a radiotherapist or a medical oncologist, and that probably fewer than 5% were entered into large multicentre randomised clinical trials. In spite of this, medical oncologists entered 57% of their patients into randomised or non-randomised, single centre or multicentre trials, and radiotherapists 15%; and 76% of oncologists and 72% of radio-therapists reported that the results of trials had influenced their clinical practice.

In this chapter we illustrate the important role that randomised trials are playing in identifying appropriate treatment policies in the management of advanced small cell and non-small cell lung cancer. In view of the benefits of such trials, recognised by oncologists and radiotherapists, a far higher proportion of patients than is currently the case should be offered the chance to participate, provided that trials continue to address clinically important issues. A major feature of some of the recent and current trials in advanced disease is that they compare not only the duration of survival with different treatment policies but also the adverse effects of treatment, the palliation of symptoms, performance status, and other aspects of quality of life. They show that much can still be done to improve the quality of survival of patients with advanced disease and a poor performance status.

Small cell lung cancer

The role of chemotherapy

With the use of combination chemotherapy, the median survival from diagnosis can be extended from three to 15 months in patients with unresectable disease that is considered to be confined to the soft tissues of one hemithorax and the ipsilateral and contralateral scalene, lower cervical, and mediastinal lymph nodes (limited disease). The median survival can be extended from less than a month to 10 months in those with more advanced, extensive disease.[23] Nevertheless, in spite of the improvements in survival to which randomised trials have led, the chances of cure remain obstinately low; the overall two year survival is generally less than 10% in a mixed population of patients with limited and extensive disease.

In view of the low cure rates, some clinicians take the view that the use of chemotherapy is not always justifiable because of toxicity and the adverse effects of treatment. They argue that there is no justification for inflicting such treatment on old and ill patients— treatment that will last for a substantial part of their remaining survival period. It is far better to keep them out of hospital and to give only non-specific palliative treatment with such agents as analgesics, antibiotics, bronchodilators, and corticosteroids, although radiotherapy or minimal chemotherapy may occasionally also be used in an attempt to relieve symptoms. The justifications for this policy are that it avoids deaths related to treatment and causes less distress, even though the duration of survival may be shorter than if a more active policy is adopted. But this approach overlooks the necessity of obtaining good control of the disease to relieve symptoms.

The MRC Lung Cancer Working Party started to address this problem in a trial of patients with either limited or extensive disease, but with good performance status. They were randomly allocated either to a policy of immediate intravenous multidrug chemotherapy or to a policy of selective treatment. In this latter group, patients were not necessarily given immediate chemotherapy or radiotherapy. Instead, treatment was given as and when required to control symptoms. The responsible clinician decided what treatment to give, but if chemotherapy was considered desirable intravenous cyclophosphamide at intervals of three weeks was recommended.[4] The most important finding from this trial was that with the policy of immediate treatment, survival was substantially longer (figure 1). Quality of life was assessed by the clinicians, who reported on adverse effects, performance status, and degree of breathlessness, and by the patients themselves, who kept a daily record on nausea and vomiting, physical activity, mood, anxiety, and overall condition, using a diary card.[5] In the light of more recent experience the working party now considers that these instruments provided an inadequate assessment of quality of life—insufficient data were collected on symptom control and psychological distress, for example. In the event the findings on quality of life were somewhat conflicting. They showed that with the policy of immediate chemotherapy, adverse effects were more common; other aspects of quality of life were better in the clinicians' assessments but worse in the patients' assessments. This trial was nevertheless important because it showed that a regimen of chemotherapy given on an outpatient basis—that is,

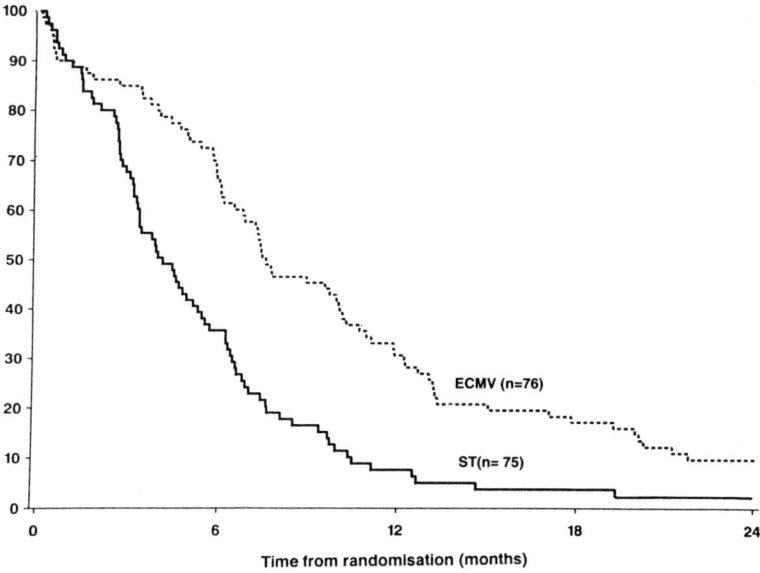

Figure 1 Percentage of patients surviving from date of randomisation in a trial comparing immediate chemotherapy with etoposide, cyclophosphamide, methotrexate, and vincristine (ECMV) with selective palliative treatment (ST) given as and when required to control symptoms. This trial showed that immediate multidrug chemotherapy is associated with a major improvement in the duration of survival without worsening quality of survival.

one of only moderate intensity—could have a major impact on survival, compared with a purely palliative policy, without significantly worsening the *quality* of survival. It drew attention to the need to study prognostic factors more closely and to determine more clearly which patients might benefit most from intensive specialised treatment and which from a more palliative approach.

Treatment policies in different prognostic groups

Analysis of routine clinical, radiographic, haematological, and biochemical data from almost 4000 patients with small cell lung cancer in United Kingdom clinical trials from eight major centres[6] showed that the best pretreatment indicators of prognosis are performance status, extent of disease, and the plasma alkaline phosphatase activity. Aspartate aminotransferase and lactate dehydrogenase activities were also useful but were not measured by all centres. Thus expensive staging such as CT and other scanning procedures are usually unnecessary and do not substantially help in separating patients into different prognostic groups.

It is becoming increasingly widely accepted that in patients with a good performance status, whether their disease is limited or extensive, tumour control is a realistic medium term goal and they should be offered multidrug chemotherapy (together with thoracic radiotherapy for those with limited disease). In patients with a poor performance status, less toxic palliative chemotherapy should be considered.[7]

Duration of chemotherapy in patients with good performance status

If the tumour responds to chemotherapy, the maximum response, complete or partial,[8] is usually achieved after only two or three courses. Several randomised trials have therefore attempted to determine the minimum number of courses of chemotherapy that can be given without compromising survival, the aim being to reduce toxicity and improve the quality of life in patients with either limited or extensive disease. In an MRC trial 265 patients responded to initial chemotherapy with six courses of etoposide, cyclophosphamide, methotrexate, and vincristine (ECMV) and were then allocated at random to receive a further six courses of the same chemotherapy (maintenance chemotherapy) or no further chemotherapy until relapse.[9] There was no overall survival advantage in either group.

In a similar trial conducted by the Midlands Small Cell Lung Cancer Group[10] 93 patients who responded to induction chemotherapy with six courses of vincristine, doxorubicin, and cyclophosphamide were allocated at random to receive a further eight courses of maintenance chemotherapy or no further chemotherapy until relapse. Maintenance chemotherapy significantly prolonged survival in patients with extensive disease on admission, but in patients with limited disease survival was longer in the group with no maintenance, although this difference was not significant.

The London Lung Cancer Group allocated 616 patients at random to receive either four or eight courses of etoposide, cyclophosphamide, and vincristine.[11] In both these groups there was a second randomisation to receive either symptomatic treatment or further chemotherapy with methotrexate and doxorubicin at relapse. The only difference was that survival was significantly shorter in patients allocated to receive four courses of initial chemotherapy without further chemotherapy on relapse.

In a trial undertaken by the EORTC,[12] 434 patients who responded to initial chemotherapy with five courses of cyclophosphamide, doxorubicin, and etoposide were allocated at random to receive conservative treatment only or a further seven courses of the same chemotherapy. There was no survival advantage in either group.

In a current MRC trial,[13] 458 patients were allocated at random to either three or six courses of ECMV or to six courses of etoposide and ifosfamide. There was no significant survival advantage for any of the three treatment groups, but the data are consistent with the possibility of lower death rate by up to 10% with the six course regimen compared with the three course regimen.

In the light of all these findings we can conclude that in terms of survival six courses of chemotherapy should be accepted as the maximum.[14] Even so, the MRC comparison of six and three courses shows that three are at most marginally less effective than six.

Palliative chemotherapy

In a study of chemotherapy as palliative treatment by the London Lung Cancer Group,[15] the patients were randomised to receive their chemotherapy either in the standard way every three weeks or only as required to reduce symptoms associated with tumour or radiological progression of disease. The hope was that the patients in this group would require less chemotherapy and therefore enjoy better quality of life. In the event less chemotherapy was indeed given to this group but palliation of symptoms was substantially less effective and quality of life was worse, showing that good control of disease and good palliation go together. In a recent MRC chemotherapy trial,[16] clinicians reported not only on the adverse effects of treatment but also on patients' symptoms, overall condition, and level of physical activity, and the patients completed a diary card. This trial also showed how effective chemotherapy is at palliating the symptoms of lung cancer (table I).

We still need to determine what types of regimen are most appropriate for patients with extensive disease and poor performance status. If chemotherapy is too intensive there is a risk of early

TABLE I   Palliation of main symptoms, as assessed by clinicians, in randomised trial of ECMV* and etoposide and ifosfamide†

Symptom	Regimen	Number of patients with symptom pretreatment	Per cent of patients with palliation	Per cent of patients in whom symptom disappeared
Cough:	ECMV3	140	80	65
	ECMV6	126	74	65
	EI6	115	83	76
Haemoptysis:	ECMV3	57	89	89
	ECMV6	44	91	89
	EI6	37	86	86
Chest pain:	ECMV3	77	86	83
	ECMV6	63	87	82
	EI6	71	82	76
Breathlessness:	ECMV3	125	58	41
	ECMV6	124	56	36
	EI6	112	71	51
Anorexia:	ECMV3	81	78	72
	ECMV6	74	76	72
	EI6	72	79	75
Dysphagia:	ECMV3	8	63	63
	ECMV6	15	80	73
	EI6	11	73	73

*Three courses (n = 157) or six courses (n = 152)
†EI for six courses (n = 149)

death associated with treatment.[9][13][17] The MRC has recently completed an intake of 310 patients with poor prognosis into a randomised trial comparing ECMV and just etoposide and vincristine (EV). Interim results suggest that survival and palliation of symptoms are similar in the two groups but that haematological toxicity was substantially less in the group receiving EV. The MRC have recently started intake into a trial comparing oral etoposide and standard multidrug intravenous chemotherapy (protocol LU16). In these trials the quality of life instruments include the Rotterdam Symptom Checklist[18] and the Hospital Anxiety and Depression Scale[19] (see chapter 10). The patient diary card used is illustrated in figure 2. It is important to include quality of life endpoints in trials of palliative treatment, bearing in mind that quality of life is a multidimensional concept that includes palliation of symptoms, adverse effects of treatment, physical wellbeing, and psychosocial factors. Comparisons of such endpoints need to be made in randomised trials because they may have an important bearing on treatment policies, and the results can be unexpected.[15][20]

Non-small cell lung cancer

Radical radiotherapy in inoperable disease

Only a small proportion of patients with inoperable non-small cell lung cancer present for treatment with disease confined to the chest, without evidence of distant spread, and with good performance status. The value of radical radiotherapy in such patients is controversial.[21] A substantial proportion of such patients treated with radiotherapy die from primary tumour without evidence of distant metastases. There is therefore a strong case for trying to improve local control.

A conventional course of radiotherapy with curative intent will usually be given in daily fractions, five days a week, over a period of up to seven weeks. But there is evidence from cell kinetic studies that tumours may then repopulate in the intervals between treatment. Non-randomised phase II studies have therefore investigated the feasibility of giving accelerated radiotherapy in which the duration of a course is reduced to limit the opportunity for regrowth. To maintain tissue tolerance, the radiotherapy has to be hyperfractionated—given in two or more fractions a day. An acceptable regimen of CHART (continuous hyperfractionated

111

CONFIDENTIAL

Patient diary card

Name..

Hospital number....................................

Doctor in charge....................................

Next appointment:

Date...

Time ....

	This column to be completed once only, before any treatment starts Date:	WEEK 1 Mon	Tue	Wed	Thur	Fri	Sat	Sun
Loss of appetite								
Nausea (feeling sick)								
Vomiting								
Cough								
Coughing up blood								
Chest pain								
Shortness of breath								
Difficulty swallowing								

Please give details of any other health problems here:

Please remember to bring this card with you at your next appointment.

If you can't keep your next appointment then continue to use the spare card, if you have one, and if possible post your completed card to us.

INSTRUCTIONS

Please complete every evening after your last meal, even when you are in hospital, by writing the number of your answer in the appropriate box, as follows:

0 — Not at all 2 — Moderately
1 — A little 3 — Very much

Figure 2 The patient diary card used in current MRC trials. Using a simple coding system, patients make a daily record of the severity of physical symptoms. Each card covers a period of five weeks. Cards are used during periods when substantial day to day changes in symptoms are expected.

accelerated radiotherapy) has now been devised and is currently being compared with conventional radical radiotherapy in a randomised trial. Patients with locally advanced non-small cell lung cancer can be offered randomisation into this trial.

Palliative radiotherapy

At present, only a small proportion of patients with inoperable non-small cell lung cancer are cured by radiotherapy. Most present with tumour too advanced for radical radiotherapy, but require palliative treatment for major symptoms related to intrathoracic tumour. Such patients are usually treated either at first presentation or, more commonly, when significant symptoms develop, with a course of palliative thoracic radiotherapy. In the United Kingdom, until very recently, a typical course would be 30 Gy in 10 fractions over two weeks.[22] This is now changing as a result of two consecutive randomised trials on palliative radiotherapy conducted by the MRC Lung Cancer Working Party.[23 24]

In the first of these trials 369 patients with their main symptoms related to the primary intrathoracic tumour were allocated at random to the conventional multifractionated regimen—30 Gy in 10 fractions (or 27 Gy in six) given daily except at weekends—or 17 Gy in two fractions of 8·5 Gy one week apart, a regimen that was already being piloted in a few centres. As assessed by the clinicians, the main thoracic symptoms of cough, haemoptysis, chest pain, breathlessness, and anorexia were palliated in high proportions of patients in both treatment groups, haemoptysis, chest pain, and anorexia disappearing for a time in well over half the patients with these symptoms (table II). Because of the high attrition rate due to death, duration of palliation was measured as the proportion of survival time during which a symptom was palliated. For all the main symptoms the median duration of palliation was 50% or more of survival. As assessed daily by the patients using a diary card, the quality of life deteriorated slightly during treatment but then improved steadily during the next five weeks. The proportion of patients with dysphagia increased considerably during treatment, but fell to the pretreatment level during the next two weeks. All these results were very similar in the two treatment groups, but there was one case of suspected radiation myelopathy in the group given two fractions. Performance status on admission had a major prognostic effect, but there was no difference in survival between the two randomised groups.

TABLE II Palliation of main symptoms as assessed by clinicians in randomised comparative trial of two fraction (F2) and standard multifractionated (FM) regimen of palliative radiotherapy in inoperable non-small cell lung cancer

Symptom	Regimen	Number of patients with symptom pretreatment	Per cent of patients with palliation	Per cent of patients in whom symptom disappeared	Median per cent of survival time in palliation
Cough:	F2	172	65	37	50
	FM	169	56	37	50
Haemoptysis:	F2	85	81	79	76
	FM	87	86	84	84
Chest pain:	F2	102	75	67	64
	FM	106	80	74	50
Breathlessness:	F2	122	66	17	50
	FM	133	57	10	50
Anorexia:	F2	107	68	58	50
	FM	106	64	58	50

We can conclude from this trial that the two fraction regimen is preferable because it is as effective as the 10 fraction regimen, but far more convenient for patients, and it uses much less machine time. Many radiotherapists have now adopted this policy.[125]

In the second trial the two fraction regimen was compared with a single fraction of 10 Gy. The 235 randomised patients were similar to those in the first trial except that intake was restricted to patients with a poor performance status, because this was known from the first trial to affect the duration of survival, and in patients with a better status a higher dose more fractionated regimen, aimed not only at palliation but also at prolonging survival, could be preferable.

Again, the levels of palliation were high and similar in the two groups and, for all the main symptoms, the duration of palliation was 50% or more of survival. On daily assessment by patients using a diary card, there was substantially less dysphagia in the group given one fraction (figure 3). This difference was not evident from the clinicians' assessments, indicating the sensivitity of the diary card in detecting day to day changes. Radiation myelopathy occurred in one of the patients given two fractions.

As a result of this trial the single fraction 10 Gy regimen is now also being used routinely.[125] It is particularly recommended for frail and ill patients with a poor prognosis, in whom it can achieve considerable palliation with minimum inconvenience.

As indicated above, many radiotherapists consider that in patients with inoperable, non-metastatic non-small cell lung cancer that is too advanced for radical radiotherapy, but with a good performance status, a more intensive regimen than one of these palliative regimens could be preferable. The MRC Lung Cancer Working Party has just completed intake of 509 such patients into a randomised trial comparing the palliative two fraction regimen and 39 Gy in 13 fractions five days a week. As assessed by the clinicians, the regimens had a similar palliative effect. As assessed by the patients using the diary card, dysphagia related to treatment was worse in the group given 39 Gy. The currently available data suggest that there could be a survival advantage for the group given 39 Gy; it will be important to establish whether this is sustained on longer follow up. To date, only one patient (in the 39 Gy group) has experienced cord damage.

There is another large group of patients who do not fall into the

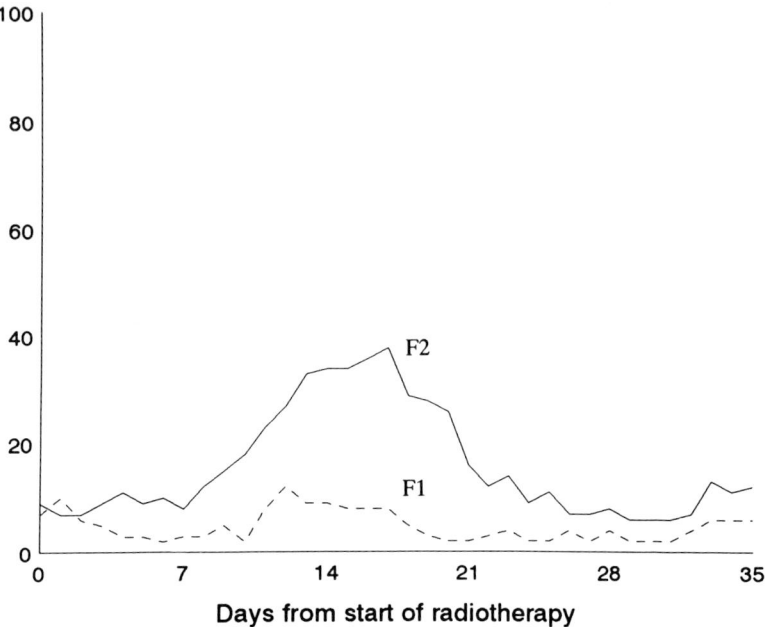

Days from start of radiotherapy

Figure 3 Percentage of patients reporting dysphagia using a diary card in a randomised trial comparing the two fraction (F2) with a single 10 Gy fraction (F1) regimen of palliative radiotherapy in inoperable non-small cell lung cancer. Clinicians assessed the patients at days 0 and 28. The F1 regimen caused substantially less dysphagia, a difference that was not detected by the clinicians in their assessments.

categories entered into the above trials. These are the patients with inoperable lesions but who have no or only minimal symptoms. There is considerable doubt as to whether such patients would benefit from immediate thoracic radiotherapy. Some clinicians advocate immediate radiotherapy in the belief that local tumour control is likely to prolong survival, improve quality of life, and prevent, delay, or improve thoracic symptoms. In sharp contrast, others argue that there is no evidence that such is the case and recommend that radiotherapy be held in reserve until needed for palliative symptom control. The MRC Lung Cancer Working Party is therefore conducting a randomised trial comparing these two approaches to management (protocol LU17).

Endobronchial treatment

Whatever the extent of non-small cell lung cancer, major obstruction of the trachea or of a main or lobar bronchus may need to be relieved. In an emergency rapid mechanical relief may be essential, but in less urgent circumstances relief may be attempted either with external beam radiotherapy—still the standard treatment in many centres—or with newer endobronchial techniques, particularly laser vaporisation, brachytherapy, or cryotherapy. There is now a need to compare the advantages and disadvantages of external beam radiotherapy with endobronchial treatment. The MRC Lung Cancer Working Party is therefore conducting such a randomised trial (protocol LU18).

Chemotherapy and immunotherapy

It is currently unclear whether adding chemotherapy or immunotherapy to other treatment modalities can improve patients' survival. Some randomised trials have attempted to find this out, but their results have been inconclusive because no individual trial has been large enough to detect a modest, but nevertheless clinically worthwhile, improvement. In fact, the results of these completed trials could be consistent with survival benefits in the region of 5–10%. Given the high incidence of non-small cell lung cancer, an improvement of only 5% would prolong the lives of thousands of people throughout the world in a year.

The most effective way to establish whether there is any reliable evidence of such survival benefits attributable to chemotherapy or immunotherapy is to undertake a systematic quantitative overview (meta analysis). This involves assembling and analysing updated data from all patients in all relevant randomised trials.[26] Such an overview is currently being conducted jointly by the MRC Cancer Trials Office, the Institut Gustave Roussy in France, and the Istituto Mario Negri in Italy. There are 58 chemotherapy trials involving more than 9000 patients, and 15 immunotherapy trials involving more than 3000 patients. Results should be available by the end of 1993.

Conclusions on non-small cell lung cancer

The above studies cover all aspects of treatment policy in the management of inoperable non-small cell lung cancer with the arguable exception of patients with inoperable stage IIIA (T$_{1-2}$,

N2, M0, or T3, N0–2, M0) disease in whom neoadjuvant chemotherapy might render a proportion resectable: trials are needed to address this issue (MRC outline protocol LU20). The results of this series of studies, when complete, will give clinicians clear guidelines for managing this common disease.

Protocols

Copies of the LU16, LU17, LU18, LU20 and CHART protocols can be obtained from the MRC Cancer Trials Office, 5 Shaftesbury Road, Cambridge CB2 2BW. Telephone: 0223 311110.

1 Stephens RJ, Gibson D. The impact of clinical trials on the treatment of lung cancer. *Clin Oncol* (in press).
2 Leonard RCF. Small cell lung cancer. *Br J Cancer* 1989;59:487–90.
3 Thatcher N, Lorrigan P, Burt P, Stout R. Intensive combined modality therapy in small cell lung cancer. *Semin Oncol* 1993; (in press).
4 Medical Research Council Lung Cancer Working Party. Survival, adverse reactions and quality of life during combination chemotherapy compared with selective palliative treatment for small-cell lung cancer. *Respir Med* 1989;83:51–8.
5 Medical Research Council Lung Cancer Working Party. Assessment of quality of life in small-cell lung cancer using a daily diary card developed by the Medical Research Council Lung Cancer Working Party. *Br J Cancer* 1991;64:299–306.
6 Rawson NSB, Peto J. An overview of prognostic factors in small cell lung cancer: a report from the Subcommittee for the Management of Lung Cancer of the United Kingdom Coordinating Committee for Cancer Research. *Br J Cancer* 1990;61:597–604.
7 Hansen HH. Management of small-cell cancer of the lung. *Lancet* 1992;339:846–9.
8 World Health Organization. *WHO handbook for reporting results of cancer treatment.* WHO Offset Publication No 48. Geneva: World Health Organization, 1979.
9 Medical Research Council Lung Cancer Working Party. Controlled trial of twelve versus six courses of chemotherapy in the treatment of small-cell lung cancer. *Br J Cancer* 1989;59:584–90.
10 Cullen M, Morgan D, Gregory W, *et al*, and the Midlands Small Cell Lung Cancer Group. Maintenance chemotherapy for anaplastic small cell carcinoma of the bronchus: a randomised controlled trial. *Cancer Chemother Pharmacol* 1986;17:157–60.
11 Spiro SG, Souhami RL, Geddes DM, *et al*. Duration of chemotherapy in small cell lung cancer: a Cancer Research Campaign trial. *Br J Cancer* 1989;59:578–83.
12 Giaccone G, Dalesio O, McVie GJ, *et al*, for the EORTC Lung Cancer Cooperative Group. Maintenance chemotherapy in small cell lung cancer: long-term results of a randomised trial. *J Clin Oncol* 1993;11:1230–40.
13 Medical Research Council Lung Cancer Working Party. A randomised trial of 3 or 6 courses of etoposide cyclophosphamide methotrexate and vincristine or 6 courses of etoposide and ifosfamide in small-cell lung cancer (SCLC) I: survival and prognostic factors. *Br J Cancer* (in press).
14 Spiro SG, Souhami RL. Duration of chemotherapy in small cell lung cancer *Thorax* 1990;45:1–2.
15 Earl HM, Rudd RM, Spiro SG, *et al*. A randomised trial of planned versus as required chemotherapy in small cell lung cancer: a Cancer Research Campaign trial. *Br J Cancer* 1991;64:566–72.
16 Medical Research Council Lung Cancer Working Party. A randomised trial of 3 or 6 courses of etoposide cyclophosphamide methotrexate and vincristine or 6 courses of

etoposide and ifosfamide in small-cell lung cancer (SCLC) II: quality of life. *Br J Cancer* (in press).

17 Morritu L, Earl HM, Souhami RL, *et al*. Patients at risk of chemotherapy-associated toxicity in small cell lung cancer. *Br J Cancer* 1989;**59**:801–4.

18 de Haes JCJ, Knippenberg FCE, Neijt JP. Measuring psychological and physical distress in cancer patients: structure and application of the Rotterdam Symptom Checklist. *Br J Cancer* 1990;**62**:1034–8.

19 Zigmond AS, Snaith RR. The Hospital Anxiety and Depression scale. *Acta Psychiatrica Scandinavica* 1983;**67**:361–70.

20 Slevin ML. Current issues in cancer—quality of life: philosophical question or clinical reality? *BMJ* 1992;**305**:466–9.

21 Saunders MI. Is control of the primary tumour worthwhile in non-oat cell carcinoma of the bronchus? *Clin Oncol* 1991;**3**:185–8.

22 Macbeth FR, Bolger J. Palliative radiotherapy for bronchial carcinoma: science or art? *Clin Oncol* 1991;**3**:245–6.

23 Medical Research Council Lung Cancer Working Party. Inoperable non-small-cell lung cancer (NSCLC): a Medical Research Council randomised trial of palliative radiotherapy with two fractions or ten fractions. *Br J Cancer* 1991;**63**:265–70.

24 Medical Research Council Lung Cancer Working Party. A Medical Research Council (MRC) randomised trial of palliative radiotherapy with two fractions or a single fraction in patients with inoperable non-small-cell lung cancer (NSCLC) and poor performance status. *Br J Cancer* 1992;**65**:934–41.

25 Maher EJ, Timothy A, Squire CJ, *et al*. Audit: the use of radiotherapy for NSCLC in the UK. *Clin Oncol* 1993;**5**:72–9.

26 Stewart LA. The role of overviews. In: Williams CJ. *Introducing new treatments for cancer: Ethical and legal problems*. Chichester: John Wiley & Sons Ltd, 1992:383–401.

8 Haematopoietic growth factors and lung cancer treatment

NICHOLAS THATCHER, HEATHER ANDERSON

Normal haematopoiesis involves a complicated but integrated process of proliferation and differentiation, with about 7×10^9 granulocytes and 1×10^{10} erythrocytes replaced hourly. The haematopoietic colony stimulating factors (CSFs) or growth factors are glycoproteins that were found to stimulate and promote the proliferation of granulocyte–monocyte progenitor cells on semisolid media in clonogenic assays (table I, figure 1). The diverse but

TABLE I   Human haematopoietic growth factors of current clinical interest*

Name	Abbreviation	Molecular weight (daltons)	Location of gene
Erythropoietin	Epo	39 000	7q 11–22
Granulocyte colony stimulating factor	G-CSF	20 000	17q 11·2–21
Granulocyte–macrophage colony stimulating factor	GM-CSF	18–30 000	5q 23–31
Macrophage colony stimulating factor	M-CSF (CSF-1)	70–90 000, 45–50 000	5q 33·1
Multipotential colony stimulating factor	Multi-CSF (IL-3)	15–30 000	5q 23–31
Interleukin-4	IL-4	16–20 000	5q 31
Interleukin-6	IL-6	19–21 000	7q 15

*Modified from Metcalf.[2]

120

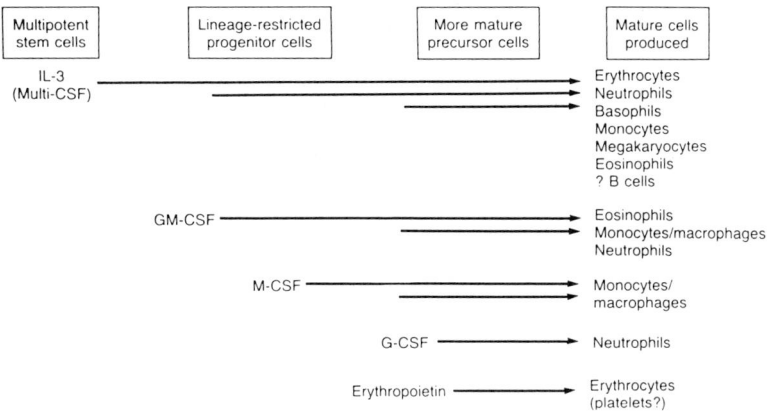

Figure 1   Targets of haematopoietic growth factors. IL-3—interleukin-3; CSF—colony stimulating factor; M–macrophage; G—granulocyte.

ordered interactions of colony stimulating factors, target cells, and stroma are responsible for the complex process of haematopoiesis. The colony stimulating factors have effects other than proliferation and differentiation, including maintenance of cell viability, membrane integrity, and functional stimulation of mature cells—for example, granulocyte phagocytosis and superoxide production (table II).[1-4]

The growth factors have very different structures and specific receptors exist on target cells, though a target cell may possess many more than one type of colony stimulating factor receptor.

TABLE II   In vitro actions of myeloid colony stimulating factors*

1   Maintain survival at all stages of development of granulocytes and monocytes
2   Presence required to induce cell division; concentration determines length of cell cycle
3   Commit bipotential granulocyte-macrophage precursor cells to enter granulocytic or monocytic lineage
4   Stimulate functional activity of mature polymorphs and monocyte-macrophages; effects on chemotaxis, expression of membrane antigens, phagocytosis, superoxide production, killing of micro-organisms and tumour cells, and production of biologically active agents (for example, interferons, tumour necrosis factor, prostaglandins)

*Modified from Steward et al.[1]

121

Growth factors are also unusual in having very high biological activity and in being able to increase rapidly given appropriate stimuli. The production of growth factors from endothelial and stromal cells, fibroblasts, lymphocytes, and macrophages is controlled by a network of interactions between the various cell types and external stimuli, such as foreign antigens and endotoxin. In addition, we are becoming increasingly aware of further important synergistic interactions between growth factors, which again emphasise the complexity of the system and the potential difficulties of full clinical exploitation.[1-6]

Various factors other than the colony stimulating factors, such as erythropoietin and the interleukins (IL), also exert effects on cellular proliferation and differentiation, with interleukins affecting B and T cell lymphocytes. Some, such as interleukin-3 (IL-3) and IL-6, also have an effect on myeloid cells (table I, figure 1). Growth factors that act on multipotent progenitor cells of early lineage—for example, IL-3—give rise to a range of mature cell types, including erythrocytes platelets, monocytes, and the various granulocytes. Granulocyte–macrophage colony stimulating factor (GM-CSF) stimulates production of granulocytes and monocytes and increases the numbers of eosinophils and lymphocytes, and, in some cases, platelets and erythrocytes, as well as neutrophils. G-CSF is much more lineage restricted and acts specifically on neutrophil granulocytes (table I, figure 1).

The genes coding for IL-3, GM-CSF, and monocyte (M) CSF are localised to a small area of chromosome 5, whereas the gene for G-CSF resides on chromosome 17 (table I). Recombinant DNA technology has enabled these factors to be further examined both in vitro and in early clinical studies. Data are now available on recombinant erythropoietin, G-CSF, and GM-CSF. Preliminary results are available for IL-3 and anticipated for IL-4 and IL-6 in the near future.

Clinical applications of growth factors in lung cancer

Haematopoietic growth factors are now the centre of feverish clinical activity in a wide range of malignant and non-malignant diseases, including solid tumours, haematopoietic malignancies, myelodysplastic syndromes, aplastic anaemia, AIDS, and the idiopathic neutropenias (table III).[1-3 6 7]

Erythropoietin

Erythropoietin has considerably improved the anaemia and quality of life in patients with end stage renal failure, provided that sufficient iron stores are present. Patients with malignant tumours, including lung cancer, often have normochromic-normocytic anaemia with a block in iron transfer from stores to the erythroid precursor cell. They may also have anaemia due to blood loss or marrow infiltration and, interestingly, the erythropoietin concentration tends to be lower in patients with malignant disease (including lung cancer) than in patients with anaemia due to other causes but of similar severity.[8 9] The erythropoietin response was also found to be decreased in patients receiving chemotherapy, though this was not due particularly to the use of nephrotoxic drugs such as cisplatin in the treatment regimen.[9] Patients with anaemia induced by chemotherapy were treated with intravenous erythropoietin in escalating dosages. No severe toxic effects were reported with doses of up to 300 IU/kg/day for five days a week for a period of four weeks. Significant increases in haemoglobin concentration after four weeks of erythropoietin at the higher doses were noted, including some patients with lung cancer who had received chemotherapy with or without cisplatin.[10 11]

An early report of a randomised study examined the effect of erythropoietin in two groups of patients and compared this with outcome in a control group.[12] All patients had small cell lung

TABLE III Potential clinical applications of myeloid colony stimulating factors*

---

1 Treatment of bone marrow failure:
   (i) idiopathic
   (ii) neoplastic
   (iii) iatrogenic
2 Augment rate of recovery after bone marrow transplantation
3 Reduce duration or degree (or both) of leucopenia following chemotherapy
4 Increase granulocyte number and function (for example, in patients with AIDS)
5 Treatment of leukaemia—altering the rates of cell reproduction and differentiation
6 Treatment of myelodysplasia—increase normal differentiation and reduce blast population
7 Treatment of established bacterial and fungal infections
8 Improve host defence against potential infection after major trauma—for example, burns

---

*Modified from Steward *et al.*[1]

123

cancer and were treated with an intensive carboplatin-ifosamide-etoposide regimen. Suppression of bone marrow made frequent blood and platelet transfusions mandatory. Erythropoietin (150 or 300 IU/kg three times a week subcutaneously) resulted in transfusion of significantly less blood in both groups receiving erythropoietin than in the control group and in a trend towards fewer platelet transfusions. The latter trend strengthens the controversial experimental observation of megakaryocyte precursor stimulation by erythropoietin. There may therefore be a case for the use of erythropoietin to reduce blood transfusions in selected patients with cancer.

Granulocyte colony stimulating factor and conventional chemotherapy

The first clinical study in patients with small cell lung cancer of a colony stimulating factor, G-CSF, was conducted in Manchester.[13] This and subsequent studies examined the effect of G-CSF after conventional dose chemotherapy in preventing drug induced neutropenia. Patients received up to six cycles of treatment with doxorubicin, ifosfamide, and etoposide and were randomised to receive G-CSF in odd (Nos 1, 3, 5) or even (2, 4, 6) cycles. The G-CSF was given by continuous 14 day intravenous infusion through an ambulatory pump, starting the day after chemotherapy. In addition, the dose-response relationship (from 1 to 40 μg/kg/day) was examined over five days before the first course of chemotherapy. The maximum response to G-CSF occurred with the 10 μg/kg/day dose and G-CSF was extremely effective in reducing severe neutropenia (defined as less than $1 \times 10^9/l$ neutrophils—a level considered to be critical as below this patients' vulnerability to life threatening infections and death from septicaemia is greatly increased). The duration of neutropenia (determined by examining the area over the curve between the actual neutrophil count and the cutoff of $1 \times 10^9/l$) was substantially reduced (median 80%) with G-CSF (figure 2). Normal or above normal neutrophil counts were obtained within two weeks of chemotherapy. Of particular importance was the observation that all six life threatening infections occurred after cycles of chemotherapy without G-CSF and no severe infection occurred after cycles in which patients were protected with G-CSF. The severe infections resulted in 30 extra days in hospital for intravenous antibiotic treatment and other supportive measures.[13]

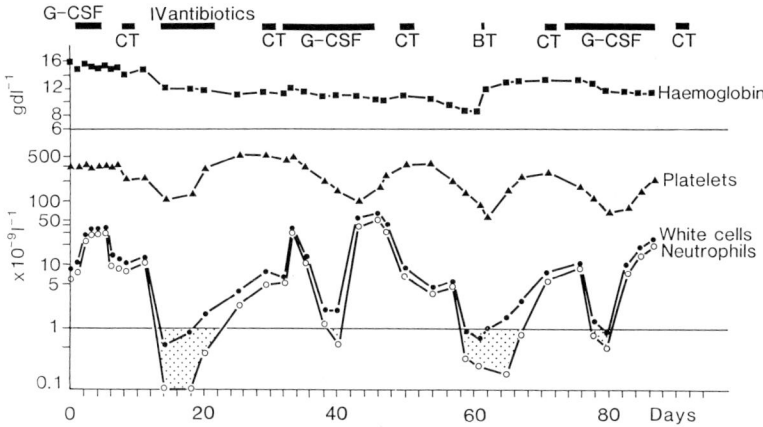

Figure 2 Haematological response to granulocyte colony stimulating factor (G-CSF) showing changes before chemotherapy (CT) and after four cycles. IV—intravenous; BT-blood transfusion. The shaded area indicates the total area of absolute neutropenia.

Other studies have confirmed these observations, particularly the specific effect on neutrophils and the fact that no toxic effects, or only very minor side effects, occurred with G-CSF. Gabrilove investigated patients with advanced transitional cell bladder cancer receiving doxorubicin, cisplatin, vinblastine, and methotrexate chemotherapy who had a short intravenous infusion of G-CSF over 30 minutes.[14] They found a reduction in the number of days of neutropenia (less than 1×10^9 neutrophils/l), and all patients were able to receive the planned chemotherapy on day 14, compared with only 29% in courses with no protection from G-CSF. Interestingly, there was also a reduction in mucositis. These investigations suggested the possibility of accelerated chemotherapy, with courses given at two week rather than the conventional three or four week intervals.

In a randomised double blind placebo trial in 126 patients with small cell lung cancer reported by Crawford, patients were given conventional doses of cyclophosphamide, doxorubin, and etoposide and randomised to receive G-CSF or no G-CSF on days 8–13 of a three week treatment cycle.[15] G-CSF was given as a subcutaneous bolus of 230 µg/m²/day. There was a significant reduction in the incidence and duration of neutropenia and in the incidence

125

of severe infection as manifest by febrile neutropenia (absolute neutrophil count of $<1 \times 10^9/l$, temperature $\geqslant 38 \cdot 2°C$). Benefit occurred both in the first cycle of chemotherapy, when deaths from infection in patients with small cell lung cancer receiving chemotherapy appear to be predominant, and in subsequent cycles. The number of days spent in hospital and receiving intensive antibiotic treatment was 40–50% less in patients treated with G-CSF. Three patients from each treatment group died as a result of infection.

A similar study has been performed in Europe (without crossover to G-CSF in the group given placebo) with the same combination of drugs. Preliminary results indicate a reduction in febrile neutropenia with a protective effect extending through all six cycles of chemotherapy, and a substantial reduction in the time spent in hospital with infections. Six per cent of patients receiving placebo died from infection. Furthermore, when observed over all six cycles of chemotherapy, 51% of patients given placebo required a reduction in chemotherapy dose compared with only 24% of patients given G-CSF.[16]

Another group of investigators, in Australia, compared the response to G-CSF given by short bolus intravenous injections, subcutaneous bolus, and subcutaneous infusion at various doses.[17 18] G-CSF again reduced the duration of neutropenia after melphalan chemotherapy, though patients previously given chemotherapy or radiotherapy did not appear to respond as well to G-CSF as did untreated patients. When G-CSF was given subcutaneously to 31 patients, including nine with lung cancer, it was again very well tolerated and substantially reduced the neutropenia, even when G-CSF was started several days after the melphalan. As in other studies using G-CSF, there were no changes in the counts of cells other than neutrophils. A dose of $3\,\mu g/kg/day$ produced similar increases in neutrophil counts when given by bolus and by continuous subcutaneous infusion, the neutrophils increasing within 24 hours with both routes.[17] In a Japanese phase I/II study of 33 patients with primary lung cancer of all histological types various chemotherapy regimens were used.[19] The optimal dose of G-CSF in these patients was $100–200\,\mu g/m^2$ given as a 30 minute intravenous infusion over 14 days; $400\,\mu g/m^2$ was recommended for patients who had had previous chemotherapy, because the bone marrow response would be impaired.[19]

Not surprisingly there is increasing interest in using CSFs with chemotherapy for advanced non-small cell lung cancer. Preliminary results with platinum combination chemotherapy and G-CSF indicate a reduction in neutropenia and the feasibility of shortening the cycle schedule as blood counts had recovered by day 14.[20][21]

GM-CSF (granulocyte macrophage colony stimulating factor) and conventional chemotherapy

In the first published clinical trial with intravenous GM-CSF patients with AIDS and bone marrow failure showed a dose dependent increase in circulating leucocytes, most being mature granulocytes. The subject has been reviewed recently.[47][22] In this and other studies peripheral eosinophilia was a feature. The stimulation of all types of granulocytes is a feature of GM-CSF, whereas G-CSF specifically stimulates neutrophil granulocytes. Combinations of GM-CSF with zidovudine are now under investigation in patients with AIDS to improve tolerance to zidovudine and reduce requirements for antibiotics. In some patients with myelodysplastic syndromes an increase in platelet and reticulocyte counts and a reduction in transfusion requirements have been observed.[1][47][22]

In 1989 some phase I studies investigated routes of administration and the GM-CSF dose-response relationship in patients with refractory, advanced solid tumours, many of whom had been treated previously. In another study from Manchester a dose-response relationship was observed with GM-CSF, with significant increases in total leucocyte, neutrophil, and eosinophil counts.[23] Of particular interest was one patient who had received a large amount of previous treatment for liposarcoma, in whom a 50% reduction of the tumour occurred after GM-CSF; the response lasted for six months. Seven other patients, with tumours that were progressing, were stabilised.[23] Further investigation of the potential anticancer activity of GM-CSF (possibly mediated through the macrophage system) is warranted. Leucocytosis, largely due to an increase in granulocytes was also reported with subcutaneous GM-CSF given once daily (3–15 µg/kg/day).[24] Thus GM-CSF is an effective stimulator of haemotopoiesis with a role in reducing cytopenia after chemotherapy and bone marrow transplantation.[1][47][22-25]

A study of GM-CSF in small cell lung cancer from Manchester had the same design as that of Bronchud et al—that is, randomisation between odd and even cycles of chemotherapy.[13][26] With subcutaneous GM-CSF given in 33 cycles intravenous antibiotics were required on six occasions for febrile neutropenia, a proportion similar to the seven out of 33 cycles without GM-CSF. Despite the reduction in neutropenia after chemotherapy the incidence of infection and requirement for intravenous antibiotics were very similar, indicating the need to examine all these clinical measures in studies of the efficacy of haemopoietic growth factors.[26] A large trial of GM-CSF in small cell lung cancer was conducted by the South West Oncology Group. Patients with limited disease were given etoposide, cisplatin, and concurrent chest radiation and randomised to receive subcutaneous GM-CSF 250 $\mu g/m^2$ twice a day for days 4–14 of each cycle. Entry to the study was closed after 213 patients had been treated because severe toxicity was seen with seven episodes of dyspnoea, respiratory infection, or pneumonitis in those given GM-CSF; there were no such episodes in the controls. Patients receiving GM-CSF had less neutropenia but there were more infections, more days with fever, and a significant increase in thrombocytopenia. The major difference between this and other studies was the concurrent use of radiotherapy and the low degree of neutropenia after the modest doses of chemotherapy.[27]

Pharmacology and toxicity

The qualitative effects of G-CSF and GM-CSF on peripheral blood neutrophils are similar. Within 30 minutes of administration of the colony stimulating factor there is a transient fall in peripheral blood neutrophils followed by a rapid and substantial increase to above baseline values about five or six hours after administration. The transient depression in the count may be caused by margination to endothelial cells. Both G-CSF and GM-CSF are capable of stimulating an increase in neutrophil function. The effects of G-CSF are, of course, limited to neutrophils; GM-CSF also enhances the number and function of eosinophils, monocytes, and macrophages. The effect on macrophages may enhance their tumourcidal activity: indeed, tumour reduction has been reported in patients given GM-SCF.[23] The increase in neutrophil count with G-CSF and the leucocytosis with GM-CSF reflect demargination, accelerated release of cells from the bone marrow, and an increase in cell proliferation.[14 7 26 28] The dose dependent increases in cell count may be many times greater than the baseline count, tending to plateau from two days onwards.[14 17 18 23–25 28] For GM-CSF the increase in white cell count may be phasic, affecting both neutrophils and (to a lesser extent) eosinophils.[23] Retreatment with GM-CSF produced similar changes in the leucocyte counts but with a more rapid increase and somewhat higher peak counts.[23][24] After G-CSF or GM-CSF is withdrawn the cell counts decline rapidly and by 24–48 hours they are back to base line values. When intravenous and subcutaneous administration of G-CSF and GM-CSF were examined the increase in peripheral blood counts appeared somewhat greater with the subcutaneous route, an important practical observation.[1][4][17][23–25] The neutrophils produced in response to G-CSF have an in vitro functional capacity similar to that of baseline neutrophils.[28] Phagocytic function as reflected by chemoluminescence was not consistently enhanced with GM-CSF, although this was more noticeable with G-CSF; both factors reduced polymorph chemotaxis.[26][28]

A randomised phase II study investigated the results of varying schedules of G-CSF in patients with extensive small cell lung cancer to optimise neutrophil response. Chemotherapy comprised cyclophosphamide, doxorubicin, and etoposide. The incidence and duration of neutropenia and the severity of thrombocytopaenia were more obvious when the first dose of G-CSF was deferred (day 8 compared with days 4 and 6 after chemotherapy).[29]

In a randomised investigation of three consecutive pilot studies conducted in Germany subcutaneous GM-CSF in patients with small cell lung cancer shortened the duration of neutropenia but not the extent after a three day cycle including doxorubicin and ifosfamide. When GM-CSF was delayed to day 8 this did not affect the blood count. GM-CSF given on the same day as chemotherapy aggravated myelosuppression. When $250 \, \mu g/m^2$ GM-CSF was started on day 4 (the day after the last dose of chemotherapy) and given until day 12, the duration of leucopenia was considerably shortened and reinstitution of chemotherapy on day 15 was possible in most patients randomised to receive GM-CSF.[30] Further studies have shown the importance of starting GM-CSF by day 4; delaying until day 8 resulted in significantly longer period of neutropenia.[31] A twice daily treatment of GM-CSF every 12 hours seemed to be more effective than the same dose being delivered once daily.[32]

G-CSF has been extremely well tolerated, with only occasional bone pain and some musculoskeletal discomfort occurring with higher doses. The discomfort is mainly in the medullary areas (sternum, jaw, pelvis, back, and limbs), usually lasts for only a few hours, and does not necessarily recur with subsequent doses. G-CSF and GM-CSF have been associated with reversible increases in lactate dehydrogenase, alkaline phosphatase, liver transaminases, and uric acid and in some patients a reduction of serum cholesterol.[1-4 22 25] More severe side effects have been reported with GM-CSF but these occurred with the higher doses of phase I studies. Side effects of GM-CSF also include bone pain in some patients; fever might complicate the management of neutropenic sepsis, although the rise in temperature is usually mild and transient. A capillary leak syndrome has resulted in fluid retention with pericardial and pleural effusions, fever, arthralgia, hypotension, and renal dysfunction, but only with higher doses. Activation of inflammatory cells with overexpression of adhesion molecules resulting in aggregation of these cells, particularly in the microvasculture, may explain in part the capillary leak. Nevertheless, increases in leucocytes occur with doses of GM-CSF that are tolerable plus platelet and reticulocyte counts have been reported to improve in some studies.[1-4 22 25]

In an occasional patient considerable leucocytosis ($> 30 \times 10^9/l$) has occurred, though this is very uncommon with the dosages now recommended—for example, 5µg/kg/day G-CSF subcutaneously for 14 days or until the counts have recovered. Such severe leucocytosis resolves rapidly once the colony stimulating factor has been discontinued.

There are theoretical drawbacks to the use of growth factors, including diversion of haematopoiesis to a specific cell type with reductions in other cells lines, toxin production, and marrow hypoplasia after "badly timed" chemotherapy. Colony stimulating factors are not recommended in the 24 hours before or after conventional chemotherapy. There is also the potential for transformation with increased growth rate of malignant cells. This is potentially important as receptors for colony stimulating factors are capable, in some cases, of modulating cell proliferation in lung cancer cell lines.[33-35] In a panel of 10 small cell lung cancer lines and two non-small cell lung cancer lines, however, GM-CSF neither seemed to stimulate nor inhibit growth.[36] Similar receptors in fresh biopsy material from small cell lung cancers (J Hampson, unpublished data) have not been identified by our group.

With the growth factors currently examined there has been no evidence of late marrow failure due to "marrow exhaustion". Neither has there been evidence of the type of wasting illness seen in rodents undergoing long term administration of GM-CSF, thought to be due to excessive macrophage activation. Neutralising antibodies to the growth factors have not been detected and there have been no reports of unexpected exacerbation of malignant disease.[1 4 7 15 22–25]

G-CSF and GM-CSF for intensification of chemotherapy

The initial studies of G-CSF and GM-CSF reporting a reduction in neutropenic infections induced by chemotherapy and in antibiotic requirements and a low incidence of side effects led to the examination of growth factors in the context of dose intensification in chemotherapy. The issue is important as there is increasing evidence that dose intensification may be associated with improved response and survival in patients with various solid tumours, including lung cancer.[37]

Accelerated chemotherapy G-CSF has been used in patients with advanced breast and ovarian cancer to facilitate escalation of the dose and rate of administration of doxorubicin. Doxorubicin could be given safely only at doses of 75 mg/m² every three weeks without G-CSF but 125 and 150 mg/m² could be administered every two weeks with G-CSF, an increase in dose intensity of up to sixfold.[38] The higher dose rates were associated with a much improved rate of complete and partial response. All patients treated with the two higher doses of 125 and 150 mg/m² responded, though non-myelosuppressive toxicity, particularly epithelial damage, then became dose limiting.[38] The study emphasised that the choice of the cytotoxic drugs is critical and must take into account the potential for severe non-myelosuppressive toxicity at doses higher than the conventional ones.

In a small study by Ardizzoni, in which accelerated chemotherapy with cyclophosphamide, doxorubicin, and vincristine alternating with cisplatin and etoposide was given without dose modification, a twofold increase in dose intensity was achieved in patients with small cell lung cancer by giving GM-CSF.[39] In the German study in which GM-CSF is being used preliminary results indicate that this may allow chemotherapy to be given at two weekly intervals with a schedule of doxorubicin, ifosfamide, and vincristine alternating with cisplatin and etoposide.[30] In a small phase I trial of GM-CSF with cisplatin at a fixed dose of

35 mg/m^2 daily for three days it had been planned to increase the dose of etoposide above 200 mg/m^2 daily for three days. This proved impossible because of neutropenia associated with fever and infection, but most patients were able to receive a three week treatment cycle because of the short duration of marrow suppression.[40] Similarly, increases in the doses of etoposide and carboplatin given to patients with small cell cancer were also not feasible because of severe, life-threatening neutropenia and thrombocytopenia, especially during successive chemotherapy cycles.[31][32] A similar study has been performed in patients with advanced non-small cell lung cancer, giving them increasing doses of cisplatin, carboplatin, and etoposide with and without GM-CSF. Neutropenia limited the doses for cycles without GM-CSF; severe cumulative thrombocytopenia led to reduced doses or delays, or both, in most patients receiving three or more cycles with GM-CSF.[41]

In a randomised study of patients with extensive stage small cell lung cancer given weekly chemotherapy with and without G-CSF the CODE regimen (cisplatin, vincristine, doxorubicin, etoposide) was investigated.[42] The interim report of the first 40 patients noted that the neutrophil counts were higher, the median duration of severe neutropenia shorter, and the number of febrile episodes significantly fewer for those patients receiving G-CSF. Overall, those patients treated with G-CSF tended to have a better performance score despite the intensive nine week treatment programme. Eighty five per cent of patients in the G-CSF group received the nine cycles within 10 weeks; only 53% of the group not receiving G-CSF were able to complete treatment within 10 weeks. A significant improvement in intensity of dose was also achieved. The projected median survival is 12 months in this group of patients with extensive stage disease. The interesting point about this study of weekly chemotherapy was the ability to give the G-CSF subcutaneously (50 µg/m^2) daily throughout the treatment programme except on the day of chemotherapy.[42]

A further investigation is now being conducted in Manchester with intensive chemotherapy—with carboplatin, ifosfamide, and etoposide—in which dosages are not modified because of previous toxicity. This regimen has resulted in two year survival rates of 30% or more in patients with limited disease.[43][44] Patients are randomised to receive or not to receive G-CSF and whenever possible the chemotherapy is given at much shorter intervals than the four to six weeks usually required for this intensive regimen.

The study should identify any survival benefits that arise from dose intensification with G-CSF and show whether reduction in neutropenia is accompanied by fewer infections and other sequelae.

Dose intensive chemotherapy with and without bone marrow transplantation Repeated courses of cisplatin, etoposide, and cyclophosphamide have been given in doses for which transplantation is usually necessary to 24 patients with refractory malignancies (including some with lung cancer). G-CSF again shortened the duration of severe neutropenia in a dose related manner and enabled these patients to have fewer days of antibiotic treatment than a control group, but their length of stay in hospital was not reduced. The protective effect of G-CSF (given as a 30 minute intravenous infusion) was sustained with repeated cycles of chemotherapy.[45] In another study from Australia subcutaneous G-CSF was given to patients receiving high dose busulphan and cyclophosphamide with autologous bone marrow transplantation. Fifteen patients with non-myeloid but chemosensitive malignancies, all of whom had been previously treated with chemotherapy and some with radiotherapy, were compared with a historical control group of 18 patients who had received the same high dose treatment alone. The 15 patients had a faster neutrophil recovery than the control group (mean day 11 *v* day 20). When compared with the controls there was a fewer days of parenteral antibiotic treatment (11 *v* 18 days), and a fewer days of parenteral nutrition for severe oral mucositis (10 *v* 16 days). The number of days spent in hospital (23 *v* 30) did not differ significantly. Doses of G-CSF were decreased stepwise once the neutrophil count exceeded $1 \times 10^9/l$ for three consecutive days and needed to be reintroduced to maintain the count in only three of the original 15 patients.[46]

The use of GM-CSF after autologous bone marrow transplantation in patients with lymphoid malignancies has been reviewed.[4 25] Again there was accelerated recovery in 15 patients given treatment, not only of granulocytes but also of platelets by one to two weeks. Some survival advantage has also been claimed.[25] In patients with refractory breast cancer and metastatic melanoma given high dose treatment with cyclophosphamide, carmustine, and cisplatin followed by autologous bone marrow transplantation GM-CSF doses unassociated with substantial toxicity resulted in accelerated recovery of the total white cell count. The patients receiving GM-CSF tolerated chemotherapy with considerably less subjective and objective evidence of toxicity than the controls, with fewer episodes of septicaemia and less hepatotoxicity and nephrotoxicity, possibly as a result of fewer infections.[47] These and other studies suggest that accelerated and high dose chemotherapy, with repeated courses, are possible, and this will reopen the issue of repeated high dose treatment for chemosensitive tumours such as small cell lung cancer.

Peripheral blood progenitor cell harvesting and intensive chemotherapy Haematopoietic colony stimulating factors also have the ability to increase levels of progenitor cells in peripheral blood (PBPC). The progenitors can be harvested from the peripheral blood by apheresis and used as an adjunct to marrow cells, or possibly in place of them, for reconstitution after myeloablative treatment.[14 48–50] As an example, after high dose cyclophosphamide chemotherapy there is a 30-fold increase in peripheral blood progenitor cells during the rapid recovery phase of the drug induced pancytopenia. The increase can be augmented by GM-CSF up to a 1000-fold in some circumstances.[49–51] Collection of PBPC by apheresis by means of a cell separator, cryopreservation, and subsequent reinfusion has substantially accelerated haematopoietic reconstitution after high dose chemotherapy and radiotherapy in patients with advanced malignancy, including small cell lung cancer.[50 51] A recent trial has indicated that reinfusion of peripheral blood progenitors, mobilised by G-CSF, together with harvested marrow, significantly reduced the duration of neutropenia and thrombocytopenia compared with marrow alone.[52]

Even in patients who have not received high dose chemotherapy G-CSF and GM-CSF are capable of increasing progenitor cells of both the myeloid and the erythroid series.[48] The most dramatic result is enhanced granulocyte recovery but the number of platelet transfusions may also be reduced.[50 53] Results are available for a variety of solid tumours, most of which have been treated with chemotherapy before. PBPC were obtained by sequential harvesting and reinfusion after repeated courses of high dose carboplatin and GM-CSF. Myelosuppression, including thrombocytopenia, was significantly reduced as was the requirement for transfusions, intravenous antibiotics and time spent in hospital compared with patients receiving GM-CSF alone. The use of PBPC also led to a substantial increase (38%) in dose intensity with a 70% objective tumour response rate.[54] The increase in PBPC by colony stimulating factors may provide sufficient numbers for collection using very few aphereses. Indeed, the number of cells thought to be needed for reconstitution might be obtained from just 500 ml of whole blood taken after chemotherapy and treatment with colony stimulating factor. Such an investigation is currently underway at our institution in patients with small cell lung cancer.

Cost considerations

In the studies published to date prophylaxis with G-CSF and GM-CSF has usually been given a day after each course of chemotherapy and continued for one to two weeks. The cost of these agents for each patient over seven days is about £600. The widespread use of G-CSF or GM-CSF in patients receiving chemotherapy will limit morbidity, although not in all patients, but the cost of treatment will be massively increased. As yet no clear effect on treatment related mortality has been established. Proponents argue that part of the cost of treatment with colony stimulating factors can be offset by the small reduction in the number of days spent in hospital for febrile neutropenia. But such a cost benefit is unlikely to be realised if the bed is immediately filled by another patient. Clearly it would be important to try to identify those patients at particular risk of neutropenic sepsis from chemotherapy. Indeed, this has been attempted.[55]

Treatment with colony stimulating factors could be started at a given level of neutropenia. For example, G-CSF 5 µg/kg/day has been administered only when the absolute neutrophil count has declined to $\leqslant 1 \times 10^9/l$ and continued until one day after a rise in neutrophils to $\geqslant 1.5 \times 10^9/l$. In this preliminary investigation there were no deaths from infection, although there was a 6% complication rate from neutropenic infections.[56] The median cost of G-CSF for each patient for one course was $1515. The comparable cost for G-CSF conventionally administered on a prophylactic basis would have been $4242 per patient. Cost of care, apart from G-CSF, seemed to be similar.[56] The use of G-CSF following chemotherapy directed by the neutrophil counts might be as effective and less costly than conventional G-CSF regimens.

There is a current tendency for British drugs and therapeutics committees to extend this concept further by delaying for up to 48

135

hours the institution of G-CSF in patients with neutropenic fever who fail to respond to broad spectrum antibiotics. This practice could be risky because deaths from infection occur unexpectedly and often outside the hospital environment. Even in hospital the first few hours, let alone days, of neutropenic sepsis, are generally critical. Monitoring outpatients' daily blood counts to detect early neutropenia is currently not generally possible, but in the future some form of device for measuring the white count at home might be developed.

Another means of reducing costs might be to give very short courses of G-CSF or GM-CSF lasting only a few days. This might be as effective in correcting dangerous neutropenia as more extended administration of colony stimulating factor. Regrettably, following licensing by the regulatory authorities, such studies are now extremely difficult to perform. The cost of the colony stimulating factors prevents trials not sponsored by industry from being initiated. These considerations largely depend on the priority given to this treatment by the patient, treating hospital, or funding body. The issue of whether growth factors are better than prophylactic antibiotics at reducing febrile neutropenia associated with chemotherapy should also be studied. The randomised investigation of broad spectrum antibiotics alone compared with colony stimulating factor alone or both combined should have been undertaken before the CSFs were licensed.

The concurrent administration of colony stimulating factors with chemotherapy to allow integration into weekly or rapidly accelerated treatment programmes needs to be investigated. The use of colony stimulating factors in combined modality treatment may be not as straightforward as indicated by the recent SWOG (South West Oncology Group) study of GM-CSF, which showed unexpected toxicity in those patients given growth factor.[27] There is an increasing tendency to use colony stimulating factors to intensify the doses of chemotherapy, but again there have been no large controlled randomised trials. To demonstrate the benefits or otherwise of growth factor support the MRC Lung Cancer Working Party will mount a randomised study, including an economic evaluation of G-CSF, in patients with small cell lung cancer. A standard doxorubicin, cyclophosphamide, etoposide regimen without any reductions in dose will be given, fortnightly when possible, depending on white cell recovery.

The future

The clinical use of recombinant human haematopoietic growth factors has already led to important advances in the management of patients with cancer. Bone marrow impairment is often the dose limiting complication for chemotherapeutic agents and amelioration of the profound neutropenia and associated life threatening infections is now possible.

The optimal schedules for colony stimulating factors are still unknown and not all studies with G-CSF and GM-CSF have shown a reduction in infection. Our current administration of these growth factors is unphysiological and a periodic pulse delivery of colony stimulating factors, given the physiological example of hormone release, would perhaps be more appropriate. Nevertheless, colony stimulating factors have produced clinical effects during profound bone marrow suppression when release of growth factors is likely to be at a physiological maximum.

The recovery of haematopoietic progenitor cells from peripheral blood is likely to be of great importance in enhancing haematological recovery after myelosuppressive treatment. This may even replace marrow transplantation and its associated difficulties. Much work still needs to be performed to determine the correct timing for the harvest and to find out how to obtain the optimal number of PBPC with colony stimulating factors used alone or in conjunction with chemotherapy. Furthermore, combinations of colony stimulating factors, including G-CSF and GM-CSF, with other growth factors, such as IL-3, cause synergistic effects in animal models.[5] Interleukin 3 alone has already been examined in a phase I study in patients with relapsed small cell lung cancer who were treated with vincristine, ifosfamide, and carboplatin. Interleukin 3 at higher doses ($\geqslant 8$ µg/kg) significantly accelerated recovery of leucocyte and neutrophil counts and increased numbers of monocytes and eosinophils. The numbers of reticulocytes and platelets also increased. Interleukin 3 has also been safely administered after chemotherapy in outpatients.[57] The combinations are potentially capable of restoring all aspects of haematopoiesis after marrow suppression more rapidly than a single colony stimulating factor.[5] Initial data from clinical studies certainly seem to support this.[5] IL-6 is of particular interest as it has a considerable effect on megakaryocytes and may well diminish thrombocytopenia. The introduction of megakaryocytic colony stimulating factor and thrombopoietin also is eagerly awaited for overcoming thrombocytopenia. Treatment with IL-3 followed by GM-CSF after etoposide, ifosfimide, and cisplatin produces a manyfold increase in the number of progenitor cells within a few days of administration.[5] Such combinations should improve the yield of peripheral blood cells for marrow rescue after repeated courses of intensive treatment in the future. There is also the possibility of obtaining sufficient numbers of progenitor cells by venesection, and thus avoiding the logistic difficulties of apheresis.

Further clinical exploitation of combinations of growth factors is likely to follow in the very near future. It would seem reasonable, for example, to use IL-6 to stimulate primitive stem cells followed by IL-3 to augment multipotent progenitors and GM-CSF to improve myelopoiesis. These would be followed by other factors, such as G-CSF or erythropoietin to act on more mature precursor cells. This type of schedule might lead to maximum stimulation and more rapid recovery of all cell types after marrow suppression.

Synthetic materials also help to protect against myelosuppression and other forms of toxicity induced by chemotherapy. Ethyol WR2721 was developed as a radioprotective drug and is taken up differentially by normal rather than malignant cells. Some clinical studies indicate that ethyol can protect patients against myelosuppression, neurotoxicity, and nephrotoxicity associated with cyclophosphamide and cisplatin, an approach also worthy of further investigation.[58 59]

Some growth factors, such as GM-CSF, IL-4, and IL-6, modify the cell cycle. GM-CSF shortens the total cycle and the duration of the S phase of bone marrow cells. Once GM-CSF is stopped the rate of marrow proliferation falls dramatically to below the pretreatment rate. Scheduling cytotoxic drugs, with GM-CSF to reduce myelotoxicity, is another interesting prospect particularly for drugs that are cell cycle specific. If haematopoietic growth factors and interleukins are required for growth of malignant cells (for example, IL-6 for the myeloma cell) via autocrine or paracrine loops, inhibitors of these factors may be of value. GM-CSF and other factors may have antitumour effects in their own right by enhancing the activity of myeloid cells and inducing release of cytokines (such as interferons) that are capable of tumour cell killing. Intraperitoneal GM-CSF in patients with ovarian cancer is currently being assessed and similar consideration could be given to malignant pleural effusions in patients with mesothelioma.

Another new approach would be to use inhibitors of haematopoiesis with cancer chemotherapy. Several short (3–5) chain amino acid peptides inhibit cell proliferation and some inhibit normal haematopoiesis. Such inhibitors, when clinically available, could protect the bone marrow by reducing sensitivity of the marrow to the effects of chemotherapy.

The use of recombinant DNA technology has produced a range of colony stimulating factors, which are now available for clinical study. The early results indicate that these factors substantially ameliorate some of the toxic effects of chemotherapy with conventional and even accelerated or high dose treatment. Fuller exploration of the factors currently available and those likely to be available in the near future will require some carefully designed clinical studies. We must hope not only that the colony stimulating factors will improve the safety of cancer chemotherapy but also, because they allow greater flexibility in chemotherapy, that the problems of dose intensity can be addressed and survival and other benefits examined. It is fitting that the first clinical study with a colony stimulating factor took place in oncology patients with the most common malignancy in Britain. Further studies in these and other patients are already providing very valuable information and should lead to improvements in the management of patients with other cancers. The development of recombinant haematopoietic factors is a very potent illustration of the benefit to be obtained when basic science is linked with cancer medicine.

We would like to thank Mrs Eileen Morgan for her assistance with typing.

1 Steward WP, Thatcher N, Kaye SB. Clinical applications of myeloid colony stimulating factors. *Cancer Treat Rev* 1990;**17**:77–87.
2 Metcalf D. Haemopoietic growth factors 1. *Lancet* 1989;i:825–7.
3 Metcalf D. Haemopoietic growth factors 2: clinical applications. *Lancet* 1989;i:885–7.
4 Lieschke GJ, Burgess AW. Granulocyte colony-stimulating factor and granulocyte-macrophage colony-stimulating factor. *N Engl J Med* 1992;**327**:28–35.
5 Brugger W, Bross KJ, Lindemann A, Kanz L, Mertelsmann R. Role of hematopoietic growth factor combinations in experimental and clinical oncology *Semin Oncol* 1992;**19**(suppl 4):8–15.
6 Gabrilove J. The development of granulocyte colony-stimulating factor in its various clinical applications. *Blood* 1992;**80**:1382–5.
7 Lieschke GJ, Burgess AW. Granulocyte colony-stimulating factor and granulocyte-macrophage colony-stimulating factor. *N Engl J Med* 1992;**327**:99–107.
8 Cox R, Musial T, Gyde OHB. Reduced erythropoietin levels as a cause of anaemia in patients with lung cancer. *Eur J Cancer Clin Oncol* 1986;**22**:511–14.
9 Miller CB, Jones RJ, Piantadosi S, Abeloff MD, Spivak JL. Decreased erythropoietin response in patients with the anemia of cancer. *N Engl J Med* 1990;**322**:1689–92.
10 Platanias LC, Miller CB, Mick R, *et al.* Treatment of chemotherapy-induced anemia with recombinant human erythropoietin in cancer patients. *J Clin Oncol* 1991;**9**:2021–6.

11 Miller CB, Platanias LC, Mills SR, et al. Phase I–II trial of erythropoietin in the treatment of cisplatin-associated anemia. JNCI 1992;84:98–103.

12 de Campos ES, Radford JA, Steward WP, Hill R, Thatcher N. The effect of rHu erythropoietin (Epo) on levels of haemoglobin and number of red cell and platelet transfusions during intensive chemotherapy for small cell lung carcinoma (SCLC). BACR/ACP Annual Meeting 1991 Br J Cancer 63:A10.

13 Bronchud MH, Scarffe JH, Thatcher N, et al. PhaseI/II study of recombinant human granulocyte colony-stimulating factor in patients receiving intensive chemotherapy for small cell lung cancer. Br J Cancer 1987;56:809–13.

14 Gabrilove JL, Jakubowski A, Scher H, et al. Effect of granulocyte colony-stimulating factor on neutropenia and associated morbidity due to chemotherapy for transitional cell carcinomas of the urothelium. N Engl J Med 1988;318:1414–22.

15 Crawford J, Ozer H, Stoller R, et al. Reduction by granulocyte colony-stimulating factor of fever and neutropenia induced by chemotherapy in patients with small-cell lung cancer. N Engl J Med 1991;325:164–70.

16 Green JA, Trillet VN, Manegold C. r-metHuG-CSF (G-CSF) with CDE chemotherapy (CT) in small cell lung cancer (SCLC): interim results from a randomized, placebo controlled trial. Proc Am Soc Clin Oncol 1991;10:A832.

17 Morstyn G, Campbell L, Lieschke G, et al. Treatment of chemotherapy-induced neutropenia by subcutaneously administered granulocyte colony-stimulating factor with optimization of dose and duration of therapy. J Clin Oncol 1989;7:1554–62.

18 Morstyn G, Campbell L, Souza LM, et al. Effect of granulocyte colony stimulating factor on neutropenia induced by cytotoxic chemotherapy. Lancet 1988;i:667–72.

19 Eguchi K, Sasaki S, Tamura T, et al. Dose escalation study of recombinant human granulocyte-colony-stimulating factor (KRN8601) in patients with advanced malignancy. Cancer Res 1989;49:5221–4.

20 Johnson D, Belani C, Mason B, et al. A phase II trial of recombinant human granyulocyte colony-stimulating factor (Neupogen G-CSF) as an adjunct to cisplatin and etoposide chemotherapy in locally advanced or metastatic non-small cell lung carcinoma. Proc Am Soc Clin Oncol 1992;11:A1000.

21 Mori K, Saitou Y, Tominaga K. Phase I/II study of recombinant human G-CSF (rG-CSF) in patients receiving chemotherapy of 5-day continuous infusion of cisplatin (Pi), vindesine (V) for non-small cell lung cancer (NSCLC). Proc Am Soc Clin Oncol 1992;11:A1035.

22 Groopman JE. Status of colony stimulating factors in cancer and AIDS. Semin Oncol 1990;17(Suppl1):31–7.

23 Steward WP, Scarffe JH, Austin R, et al. Recombinant human granulocyte macrophage colony stimulating factor (rhGM-CSF) given as daily short infusions—a phase I dose-toxicity study. Br J Cancer 1989;59:142–5.

24 Lieschke GJ, Maher D, Cebon J, et al. Effects of bacterially synthesised recombinant human granulocyte–macrophage colony-stimulating factor in patients with advanced malignancy. Ann Int Med 1989;110:357–64.

25 Appelbaum FR. The clinical use of hematopoietic growth factors. Semin Hematol 1989;26(Suppl3):7–14.

26 Gurney H, Anderson H, Radford J, et al. Infection risk in patients with small cell lung cancer receiving intensive chemotherapy and recombinant human granulocyte–macrophage colony-stimulating factor. Eur J Cancer 1992;28:105–12.

27 Bunn Jr PA, Crowley J, Hazuka R, Tolley R, Livingstone R. The role of GM-CSF in limited stage SCLC: a randomized phase III study of the Southwest Oncology Group (SWOG). Proc Am Soc Clin Oncol 1992;11:A974.

28 Bronchud MH, Potter MR, Morgenstern G, et al. In vitro and in vivo analysis of the effects of recombinant human granulocyte colony-stimulating factor in patients. Br J Cancer 1988;58:64–9.

29 Crawford J, Kreisman H, Garewal H, et al. A pharmacodynamic investigation of recombinant human granulocyte colony stimulating factor (r-metHuG-CSF) schedule variation in patients with small cell lung cancer (SCLC) given CAE chemotherapy. Proc Am Soc Clin Oncol 1992;11:A1005.

30 Havemann K, Klausmann M, Wolf M, Fischer JR, Drings P, Oster W. Effect of rhGM-CSF on haematopoietic reconstitution after chemotherapy in small-cell lung cancer. J Cancer Res Clin Oncol 1991;117(Suppl iv):S203–7.

31 Bishop JF, Morstyn G, Stuart-Harris R, *et al.* Dose and schedule of granulocyte macro-phage colony stimulating factor (GM-CSF) carboplatin and etoposide in small cell lung cancer (SCLC). *Proc Am Soc Clin Oncol* 1991;**10**:A820.

32 Luikart SD, MacDonald M, Herzan D, *et al.* Ability of daily or twice daily granulocyte-macrophage-colony-stimulating factor (GM-CSF) to support dose escalation of etoposide (VP-16) and carboplatin (CBDCA) in extensive small cell lung cancer (SCLC). *Proc Am Soc Clin Oncol* 1991;**10**:A825.

33 Miyagawa K, Chiba S, Shibuya K, *et al.* Frequent expression of receptors for granulocyte-macrophage colony-stimulating factor on human nonhematopoietic tumor cell lines. *J Cell Physiol* 1990;**143**:483–7.

34 Vellenga E, Biesma B, Meyer C, Wagteveld, Esselink M, de Vries EGE. The effects of five hematopoietic growth factors on human small cell lung carcinoma cell lines: Interleukin 3 enhances the proliferation in one of the eleven cell lines. *Cancer Res* 1991;**51**:73–6.

35 Avalos BR, Gasson JC, Hedvat C, *et al.* Human granulocyte colony-stimulating factor: biologic activities and receptor characterization on hematopoietic cells and small cell lung cancer cell lines. *Blood* 1990;**75**:851–7.

36 Twentyman PR, Wright KA. Failure of GM-CSF to influence the growth of small cell and non-small cell lung cancer cell lines in vitro. *Eur J Cancer* 1991;**27**:6–8.

37 Dodwell DJ, Gurney H, Thatcher N. Dose intensity in cancer chemotherapy. *Br J Cancer* 1990;**61**:789–94.

38 Bronchud MH, Howell A, Crowther D, Hopwood P, Souza L, Dexter TM. The use of granulocyte colony-stimulating factor to increase the intensity of treatment with doxorub-icin in patients with advanced breast and ovarian cancer. *Br J Cancer* 1989;**60**:121–5.

39 Ardizzoni A, Sertoli MR, Corcione A, *et al.* Accelerated chemotherapy with or without GM-CSF for small cell lung cancer: a non-randomised pilot study. *Eur J Cancer* 1990;**26**:937–41.

40 Shepherd FA, Goss PE, Rusthoven J, Eisenhauer EA. Phase I trial of granulocyte-macrophage colony-stimulating factor with high dose cisplatin and etoposide for treatment of small-cell lung cancer: A study of the National Cancer Institute of Canada Clinical Trials Group. *JNCI* 1992;**84**:59–60.

41 Jacobs E, Bick R, Figlin R. Dose intensification study of cisplatin (CDDP), carboplatin (CBDCA) and etoposide (VP-16) with and without GM-CSF (Schering) in advanced non-small cell lung cancer (NSCLC). *Proc Am Soc Clin Oncol* 1992;**11**:A1025.

42 Masuda N, Fukuoka M, Furuse K. CODE chemotherapy with or without recombinant human granulocyte colony-stimulating factor in extensive-stage small cell lung cancer. *Oncology* 1991;**49**:19–24.

43 Thatcher N, Lind M, Stout R, *et al.* Carboplatin, ifosfamide and etoposide with mid-course vincristine and thoracic radiotherapy for "limited" stage small cell carcinoma of the bronchus. *Br J Cancer* 1989;**60**:98–101.

44 Prendiville J, Radford J, Thatcher N, *et al.* Intensive chemotherapy for small cell lung cancer using carboplatin alternating with cisplatin, ifosfamide, etoposide and mid cycle vincristine and radiotherapy. *J Clin Oncol* 1991;**9**:1446–52.

45 Neidhart J, Mangalik A, Kohler W, *et al.* Granulocyte colony-stimulating factor stimulates recovery of granulocytes in patients receiving dose-intensive chemotherapy without bone marrow transplantation. *J Clin Oncol* 1989;**7**:1685–92.

46 Sheridan WP, Morstyn G, Wolf M, *et al.* Granulocyte colony-stimulating factor and neutrophil recovery after high-dose chemotherapy and autologous bone marrow trans-plantation. *Lancet* 1989;ii:891–95.

47 Brandt SJ, Peters WP, Atwater SK, *et al.* Effect of recombinant granulocyte macrophage colony stimulating factor on hematopoietic reconstitution after high dose chemotherapy and autologous bone marrow transplantation. *N Engl J Med* 1988;**318**:869–76.

48 Griffin JD. Hemopoietins in oncology: factoring out myelosuppression. *J Clin Incol* 1989;**7**:151–5.

49 Ravagnani F, Siena S, Bregni M, Sciorelli G, Gianni AM, Pellegris G. Large-scale collection of circulating haematopoietic progenitors in cancer patients treated with high-dose cyclophosphamide and recombinant human GM-CSF. *Eur J Cancer* 1990;**26**:562–4.

50 Gianni AM, Bregni M, Siena S, *et al.* Rapid and complete hemopoietic reconstitution following combined transplantation of autologous blood and bone marrow cells. A changing role for high dose chemo-radiotherapy? *Hematol Oncol* 1989;**7**:139–48.

HAEMATOPOIETIC GROWTH FACTORS

51 Gianni AM, Siena S, Bregni M, *et al*. Granulocyte-macrophage colony-stimulating factor to harvest circulating haemopoietic stem cells for autotransplantation. *Lancet* 1989; ii:580–5.
52 Sheridan WP, Begley CG, Juttner CA, *et al*. Effective peripheral blood progenitor cells mobilized by filgrastim (G-CSF) on platelet recovery after high dose chemotherapy. *Lancet* 1992;**339**:640–4.
53 Henon PR, Butturini A, Gale RP. Blood-derived haematopoietic cell transplants: blood to blood? *Lancet* 1991;**337**:961–3.
54 Shea TC, Mason JR, Storniolo AM, *et al*. Sequential cycles of high-dose carboplation administered with recombinant human granulocyte-macrophage colony-stimulating factor and repeated infusions of autologous peripheral-blood progenitor cells: A novel and effective method for delivering multiple courses of dose-intensive therapy. *J Clin Oncol* 1992;**10**:464–73.
55 Radford JA, Ryder WDJ, Dodwell D, Anderson H, Thatcher N. Predicting septic complications of chemotherapy: an analysis of 382 patients treated for small cell lung cancer without dose reduction after major sepsis. *Eur J Cancer* 1993;**29A**:81–6.
56 Lowenbraun S, La Rocca RV. Neutrophil count-directed G-CSF administration following chemotherapy (C). *Proc Am Soc Clin Oncol* 1992;**11**:A1402.
57 Postmus PE, Gietema JA, Damsma O, *et al*. Effects of recombinant human interleukin-3 in patients with relapsed small-cell lung cancer treated with chemotherapy: a dose-finding study. *J Clin Oncol* 1992;**10**:1131–40.
58 Glover DJ, Glick JH, Weiler C, Hurowitz S, Kligerman MM. WR-2721 protects against the haematological toxicity of cyclophosphamide: a controlled Phase II trial. *J Clin Oncol* 1986;**4**:584–8.
59 Glover DJ, Glick JH, Weiler C, Fox K, Guerry D. WR-2721 and high-dose cisplatin: an active combination in the treatment of metastatic melanoma. *J Clin Oncol* 1987;**5**:574–8.

9 New drugs in lung cancer

DENIS C TALBOT, IAN E SMITH

The best hope for improved treatment of lung cancer lies in the development of effective new drugs. Lung cancer remains the main cause of cancer related death in Britain, accounting for 17% of all new registered cases of cancer and 25% of cancer deaths.[1] Over 90% of patients with lung cancer die of their disease. Despite dramatic developments with cytotoxic chemotherapy for some malignancies over the past four decades, very little impact has been made on cure rate for patients with lung cancer. This is brought into perspective by comparing the change in survival rates of lung cancer and childhood acute lymphoblastic leukaemia over the past two decades. The five year survival rate for acute lymphoblastic leukaemia has increased from 8% to 70% as a result of improved treatment with cytotoxic drugs; the five year survival rate for lung cancer for all ages remains unchanged at 8%, with over 40 000 deaths each year in the United Kingdom alone.

Prospects are bleak for all histological subtypes. Small cell lung cancer is very chemosensitive in its initial clinical stages; treatment with appropriate chemotherapy does improve survival, but only to around 10–15 months for patients with limited disease and to seven to 11 months for those with extensive disease. Deaths from small cell lung cancer continue to occur beyond two years from diagnosis resulting in a dismal five year survival rate of only 2·5%.[2] For patients with non-small cell lung cancer surgery offers the best chance of cure, but by the time the diagnosis is made most patients have inoperable disease. The role of chemotherapy in the management of advanced non-small cell lung cancer is controversial.

143

Modest response rates of 25–50% are achieved with combination chemotherapy containing cisplatin, but the response usually lasts only a few months and the survival benefit is marginal.[3]

Most drugs used in the treatment of cancer have been developed by empirical means or by extensive screening. Many of the pharmacological properties of a new drug are not determined until some time after the drug has achieved wide clinical application. A fuller understanding of the biology of lung cancer may allow us to identify specific molecular targets for which to design new drugs.[4] An encouraging development is the characterisation of receptors for autocrine and paracrine growth factors for small cell lung cancer and of an increased understanding of the signal transduction. Other possible drug targets include DNA repair enzymes, the genes for tumour promoters and suppressors, tumour cell cycle regulatory genes and their products.

Small cell lung cancer

When to assess new drugs

Small cell lung cancer is one of the most chemosensitive of the solid tumours, and many drugs have activity against this form of lung cancer.[5] Much clinical research effort has gone into investigating combination chemotherapy, alternating chemotherapy, maintenance treatment and high dose chemotherapy with autologous bone marrow rescue. Yet the median survival has been prolonged by only a few months. The rapid recurrence seen in most patients after initial tumour regression indicates that the key problem is drug resistance. This points to an important question in the development of drugs: when should new drugs be assessed? The conventional approach has been to test new drugs only after conventional chemotherapy has failed. Not unexpectedly, in this drug resistant environment results are much worse than when the same agent is tested in previously untreated patients. Etoposide when given as a single agent had a response rate of 80% in untreated patients[6] but only 10% in patients previously treated with cytotoxic drugs.[7] Similarly, teniposide has a reported 90% response rate in untreated patients,[8] compared with 6% in previously treated patients.[9] Initial studies with carboplatin showed response rates of 60% for untreated patients, compared with 19% for treated patients.[10]

Testing new drugs in previously untreated patients clearly minimises the risk of rejecting a clinically useful drug because it lacks efficacy in patients with resistant disease. On the other hand, this approach is not straightforward because the survival and quality of life of the patient may be jeopardised if an inactive drug is tested in untreated patients. In a phase II trial of oral idarubicin in 21 untreated patients with extensive disease a response rate of only 14% was observed. Despite a policy of switching promptly to cyclophosphamide, vincristine, and etoposide, only 14 patients were well enough to do this and the response rate was low at 19%, with a short median survival of six months.[11] The outcome was the same in two other trials of similar design in patients with extensive disease: median survival times of only seven weeks were achieved with triglycidylurazole[12] and eight weeks with mitozantrone[13]— similar to the survival expected for untreated patients with extensive small cell lung cancer. If the agent under investigation has low activity then the patient is effectively receiving no treatment, and the chance for useful palliation with conventional chemotherapy is lost.

What, therefore, is the best way to evaluate new drugs in small cell lung cancer? An important prerequisite is for patients receiving a trial drug to have a good performance status without metastatic disease that is currently life threatening. Several methods are then possible.

The first is to add the drug under investigation to an otherwise standard combination and compare this regimen with the standard combination alone. When this method was used to evaluate cisplatin, 100 patients with extensive small cell lung cancer were randomised to receive etoposide, cyclophosphamide, doxorubicin, and vincristine with or without cisplatin. The objective response rate was 48% in the four drug combination and 83% in the five drug combination containing cisplatin.[14] This method overcomes the problem of testing drugs with low activity but has a number of disadvantages. Because most combinations now give high response rates, large numbers of patients need to be randomised in this kind of study to confirm an increase in response. Furthermore, the activity of the drug as a single agent cannot be determined by this means.

Good, albeit short-lived, response rates to second line or rechallenge chemotherapy makes the testing of new agents in patients who have relapsed once off treatment an attractive option. A

145

review of 97 phase II studies in small cell lung cancer supports this.[15] Thus a second approach would be to accept response rates of 10% or even 5%, in previously treated patients, as the threshold for further evaluation of efficacy. This might require large numbers of patients to attain satisfactory confidence limits and the power to identify active agents. A two stage sequential trial design using this approach has been proposed by Grant *et al.*[16]

A third strategy would be to randomise previously untreated patients to receive standard first line induction drugs or the phase II drug. Patients with stable or progressive disease after one or two cycles or progressive disease after an initial response would receive conventional salvage chemotherapy. This method was used in the Eastern Cooperative Oncology Group phase II study of menogaril. The standard induction drugs were cyclophosphamide, doxorubicin, and vincristine, with etoposide and cisplatin as salvage chemotherapy. Menogaril was found to be inactive in terms of the response criteria; the estimated median survival times were 42 weeks for patients receiving cyclophosphamide, doxorubicin, and vincristine and 38 weeks for those having menogaril, but the differences were not significant.[17]

A further approach would be to randomise patients to receive standard induction treatment or the study drug for a maximum of two cycles only. Patients with progressive disease after one cycle of the study drug are immediately switched to the standard combination and all other patients on the new drugs are automatically switched to standard drugs after two cycles irrespective of response. This enables the response to be appropriately evaluated and establishes whether the chance of long term survival has been reduced by treating patients with the study drug as first line therapy. Moore and Korn argue the case for evaluating new agents in previously untreated patients only in the following circumstances: (i) agents having novel or unknown mechanisms of action and having activity in other solid tumours; (ii) agents with specific activity for small cell lung cancer in pre-clinical testing; or (iii) analogues of active drugs.[18]

New drugs

Recent phase II studies of single agents are shown in table I. One of the most active agents developed recently is the water soluble semisynthetic *camptothecin analogue CPT11*. The parent molecule camptothecin is a plant alkaloid isolated from the Asian

TABLE I Clinical trials of new drugs (single agents) for small cell lung cancer

Drug	Dose and schedule	Not previously treated	Previously treated	Total No evaluable	CR	PR	Response (%)	Median duration of survival (w)	Reference
Ifosfamide	500 mg PO bd × 14 d q 28 d	NS	NS	14	1	6	50	NS	Manegold[67]
Ifosfamide	1·5 g/m² IV d × 5 q 21 d	44	0	44	4	17	48	43	Ettinger[68]
Ifosfamide	5 g/m² IV q 21 d	0	14	14	0	6	43	NS	Cantwell[31]
Epirubicin	120 mg/m² IV q 21 d	80	0	71	4	30	48	30	Eckhardt[24]
Teniposide	60 mg/m² IV d × 5 q 21 d	46	0	46	2	18	43	38	Ettinger[68]
Teniposide	120–140 mg/m² IV d 1,3,5 q 21 d	12	36	44	4	11	34	34	Giaccone[69]
CPT-11	100 mg/m² IV q 7 d	8	33	35	2	7	33	NS	Negoro[21]
Mitoxolomide	70–90 mg/m² PO q 42 d	11	9	18	0	5	28	NS	Harding[70]
Interleukin-2	3 × 10⁶ Nutley Units/m²/d IV for 96 h q 7 d*	0	73	24	5	1	25	52	Clamon[35]
Navelbine	30 mg/m² IV q w	0	26	25	0	4	16	NS	Jassem[71]
Pirarubicin	60–70 mg/m² IV q 21 d	1	13	14	0	2	14	21	Montalar[25]
Menogaril	200 mg/m² IV q 28 d	40	0	40	0	2	5	38	Ettinger[72]

*All patients given induction chemotherapy followed by interleukin-2 for patients with assessable disease not achieving CR, complete response; IV, intravenously; d, day; q, every; bd, twice daily; w, week; tiw, three times a week; PO, orally; CR, complete response; PR, partial response; NS, not stated.

147

tree *Camptotheca acuminata*. Although cimptothecin is active against experimental tumours, its clinical use is limited by severe haemorrhagic cystitis and low response rates.[19] CPT11 is a potent inhibitor of topoisomerase I, an enzyme which creates transient breaks in one strand of duplex DNA to facilitate local unwinding during DNA replication and the elongation step of transcription. It has encouraging preclinical and antitumour activity and is better tolerated than camptothecin. Phase I studies with single doses of CPT 11 have shown that it has a maximum tolerated dose of $250\,\text{mg/m}^2$, the dose limiting toxicity being myelosuppression. Other adverse reactions include alopecia and gastrointestinal toxicity but not haemorrhagic cystitis.[20] The results of the first phase II study of CPT11 in small cell lung cancer are encouraging. Forty one patients received CPT11 $100\,\text{mg/m}^2$ by intravenous infusion over 90 minutes every week, with dose reduction for neutropenia. Two of 27 previously treated evaluable patients had a complete response and seven had a partial response (objective response 33%). Of eight evaluable previously untreated patients, four had a partial response. The median duration of response was 50 days.[21] Pharmacokinetic studies of CPT11 and its active metabolic SN38 showed that elimination is triphasic, with a long terminal half life of 18 hours, clearly an advantage for a drug active in S phase.[22] Other camptothecin analogues are being evaluated, including topotecan (SKF104864), which is currently undergoing phase I clinical trials.

Much of the effort put into development of drugs for small cell lung cancer has focused on the assessment of analogues of existing active groups of drugs, notably the anthracyclines and epipodophyllotoxins. *Epirubicin* (4-epidoxorubicin) has been in clinical use for some years but more recently has been assessed in dose escalation studies in patients with solid tumours. The clinical trials group of the National Cancer Institute of Canada gave Epirubicin 100–$120\,\text{mg/m}^2$ intravenously every three weeks to patients with extensive disease. An objective response rate of 50% was achieved, with a median survival of 35 weeks.[23] Adverse effects included, predictably, moderate myelosuppression, alopecia, nausea, and vomiting but not cardiotoxicity. A similar response rate was reported by Eckhardt in 80 previously untreated patients receiving $120\,\text{mg/m}^2$ every three weeks. In this series one patient developed congestive cardiac failure, which was fatal.[24] Another analogue, 4^1-0-Tetrahydroxypyronil-doxorubicin (*Pirarubicin*) at intravenous doses of 60–70 mg/m^2 every three weeks was well tolerated by previously treated patients and resulted in partial responses in two of the 14 patients.[25]

The epipodophyllotoxin etoposide, particularly in combination, is one of the most active treatments for small cell lung cancer. As a phase specific drug acting in the G_2 phase of the cell cycle cytotoxicity is highly dependent on scheduling. Response rate and survival of patients with small cell lung cancer are substantially improved when etoposide is given as five daily infusions of 100 mg/m^2 compared with a single infusion of 500 mg/m^2.[26] Phase II studies indicate that oral etoposide has the advantages of easy administration and acceptable toxicity, although the bioavailability is highly variable.[27] Molecular modification to give predictable bioavailability would further improve its clinical usefulness.

Despite the synthesis of many new derivatives of the epipodophyllotoxins, *etoposide* and *teniposide* remain the most effective members of this class of cytotoxic agent. A Danish study comparing these agents in 103 randomised patients showed no difference in response rates or median duration of survival at doses thought to be of equivalent toxicity. Patients randomised to receive teniposide, however, had lower nadir leucocyte counts.[28] We now know more about the interaction of epipodophyllotoxins with topoisomerases and DNA. Computer assisted molecular modelling has permitted a more rational design of new topoisomerase II inhibitors such as azatoxin[29]: these are more specific and potentially more clinically effective.

Ifosfamide also appears to be well suited to combination chemotherapy in the treatment of small cell lung cancer as it is less myelosuppressive than its parent alkylating agent cyclophosphamide. Ifosfamide is active in tumours resistant to standard alkylating agents, and its dose limiting toxicity, haemorrhagic cystitis, can be abrogated by Mesna without loss of efficacy.[30] It has activity as a single agent in patients previously treated with etoposide, vincristine, and doxorubicin,[31] though response rates appear to be reduced if prior treatment includes cyclophosphamide.[32] A study using ifosfamide in combination with carboplatin and etoposide (ICE), achieved a high response rate of 94% and a median survival of 19 months. Subsequent consecutive studies, using similar regimens, have reported a two year survival rate of 30% after a minimum follow up of 24 months.[33]

Drugs containing platinum, and in particular *carboplatin*, continue to play a prominent part in the management of small cell lung cancer.[34] Phase I studies of oral third generation platinum analogues are in progress, but their clinical efficacy in small cell lung cancer has yet to be assessed. A combination of oral etoposide and platinum could potentially be used as outpatient treatment in the future.

Biological response modifiers represent a new modality in cancer treatment. Preliminary results are becoming available from studies in small cell lung cancer. A phase II trial of *interleukin-2* in extensive disease is currently in progress.[35] Previously untreated patients were initially given four cycles of doxorubicin, cyclophosphamide, etoposide, and platinum. Four weeks later all patients not achieving a complete response received a continuous infusion of interleukin-2 (3×10^6 Nutley Units/m^2 a day) for four days repeated weekly for up to eight weeks. Of 73 patients, 24 were treated with interleukin-2; six had an objective response, including five with complete remissions. Toxicity including hypotension, haemolysis, renal failure, hepatic dysfunction, and allergy was severe enough to require discontinuation of treatment in at least 20% of patients.[35] The long term role, if any, for interleukin-2 in the treatment of small cell lung cancer remains to be determined. Data from preclinical studies suggest that the interferons have an anti-tumour effect for smaller tumour burdens, indicating a possible role in adjuvant treatment. In a randomised phase III study of 410 patients who had responded to conventional adjuvant treatment, Mattson found that one, two, and five year survival rates in patients receiving interferon α were improved compared with those receiving either maintenance chemotherapy or no maintenance treatment.[36] Interferon γ, which has a greater immunomodulatory effect than interferon α, was studied in a randomised phase III study of 100 patients in complete remission after conventional combination cytotoxic chemotherapy. Patients were randomised to receive subcutaneous interferon γ (4×10^6 Units) daily for six months, or observation alone. No differences were shown in median or two year survival.[37] The European Organization for Research and Treatment of Cancer (EORTC) are currently conducting a similar but larger randomised study.

Non-small cell lung cancer

Non-small cell lung cancer is more chemoresistant than small cell lung cancer and the role of chemotherapy in its management remains controversial. Only a few cytotoxic drugs have even modest single agent activity in non-small cell lung cancer. The most active include ifosfamide, vindesine, vinblastine, mitomycin C, and cisplatin, all with average response rates of around 20%.[3] Combination chemotherapy regimens containing cisplatin achieve response rates of 30–50%, but the response is of short duration and real clinical benefit is uncertain. Consequently there is less of a problem in the timing of treatment with new drugs for patients with non-small cell lung cancer than with small cell lung cancer. It is arguable that results with conventional drugs are not sufficiently good to justify their use as orthodox treatment and therefore to offer new drugs as first line treatment in patients who are fit enough and who are anxious to have such treatment on an experimental basis.

Table II shows several new agents that have recently been tested in patients with non-small cell lung cancer. False positive results of phase II studies are often due to bias from low accrual rates and premature publication. On the other hand, drugs may be wrongly rejected on the grounds of low activity because the schedule was not optimal, as was the case for ifosfamide.[3] Several studies have been reported in recent years, carried out in both previously treated and "chemotherapy naive" patients.

Camptothecin analogues have shown considerable activity in early clinical trials. A Japanese study reports a response rate of 34% in previously untreated patients, based on data from 67 patients out of the 73 who entered the study.[38] Leucopenia, nausea and vomiting, and diarrhoea occurred in about half the patients. This group of drugs clearly warrants further clinical evaluation.

Navelbine is a semisynthetic vinca alkaloid that acts by inhibition of tubulin polymerisation. It has a long terminal half life by comparison with the other vinca alkaloids and a large volume of distribution, suggesting high tissue uptake, which is most striking in the lung. A 32% objective response rate was seen in 97 previously untreated patients evaluable for response, out of the original 102; similar response rates were seen for squamous cell carcinoma and adenocarcinoma. Of particular importance, the incidence of neuropathy (7%) was lower than with vincristine or vindesine. The dose limiting toxicity was granulocytopenia, but recovery time was short.[39] These results are encouraging and

TABLE II Clinical trials of new drugs (single agents) for non-small cell lung cancer

Drug	Dose and schedule	Not previously treated	Previously treated	Total No evaluable	CR	PR	Response (%)	Median duration of survival (w)	Reference
CPT-11	100 mg/m^2 IV q 7 d	73	0	67	0	23	34	43	Asakawa[38]
Interleukin-2 + TNFα	1×10^6 cetus U/m^2/24 h IV inf q 21 d 25–100 μg/m^2/d d 1–5 q 21 d								
Navelbine	25 mg/m^2 IV q 7 d	16	0	12	0	4	33	NS	Yang[50]
Gemcitabine	1–1.5 g/m^2 IV w × 3 q 28 d	102	0	97	0	31	32	NS	Yokoyama[39]
Gemcitabine	800 mg/m^2 IV q 7 d × 3	46	0	40	2	9	27	NS	Abratt[73]
Gemcitabine	90 mg/m^2 IV 2 × w	36	0	29	0	7	24	NS	Anderson[45]
Zeniplatin	145 mg/m^2 IV q 21 d	52	0	40	0	5	12	NS	Lund[74]
Taxol	250 mg/m^2 IV q 21 d	30	0	28	0	6	21	NS	Jones[40]
Fotemustine	100 mg/m^2 IV q 21 d	25	0	24	0	5	21	NS	Chang[75]
Carboplatin	130 mg/m^2 IV q 28 d	8	24	29	0	6	21	19	Monnier[46]
Epirubicin	150–165 mg/m^2 IV q 21 d	51	0	51	0	10	20	22	Gatzemeier[76]
Trimetrexate	8 mg/m^2 IV d × 5 q 21–28 d	63	0	63	0	12	19	26	Feld[77]
Trimetrexate	150 mg/m^2 IV q 14 d	52	18	59	0	11	19	32	Maroun[78]
Teniposide	120–180 mg/m^2 IV d 1, 3, 5, q 21 d	37	0	37	0	5	13	NS	Gesme[44]
(Glycolate-0,0')diammineplatinum (II)	100 mg/m^2 IV q 28 d	34	8	42	0	7	17	NS	Giaccone[79]
TCNU	40 mg/m^2 PO daily d 1–3 q 28 d	38	30	68	0	10	15	NS	Fukuda[80]
Pirarubicin	70 mg/m^2 IV q 21 d	38	0	37	0	5	14	22	Sorensen[48]
Iododoxorubicin	80 mg/m^2 IV q 21 d	47	0	45	0	6	13	19	Drings[81]
10-EDAM	80 mg/m^2 IV q 7 d	23	0	23	0	3	13	NS	Eberhardt[82]
4'-Deoxydoxorubicin	30–40 mg/m^2 IV q d	50	0	47	0	5	11	NS	Souhami[42]
Lonidamine	450–900 mg/d PO q 21 d	25	10	35	0	4	11	NS	Rose[83]
Lonidamine	450–900 mg/d PO q 21 d	69	0	69	0	7	10	33	Kokron[84]

TCNU-(1-(2-chloroethyl)-3-2(dimethylaminosulfonyl)-ethyl-1-nitrosourea). TNFα, tumour necrosis factor; IV, intravenously; q every; PO, orally; tiw, three times a week; CR, complete response; PR, partial response; NS, not stated.

warrant further evaluation of navelbine in combination with other drugs.

Zeniplatin is a water soluble, third generation platinum analogue active against murine tumour models and in human tumour xenografts. In preclinical studies it had a superior therapeutic dose ratio to that of cisplatin. We have given this drug to 30 previously untreated patients with advanced non-small cell lung cancer, six of whom achieved an objective response. In general, zeniplatin was well tolerated, apart from neutropenia, but one patient developed renal failure thought to be drug related.[40]

At least three new antimetabolites have activity as single agents in non-small cell lung cancer. 10-EDAM (10-ethyl-5-deaza-aminopterin) is a methotrexate analogue that has a modification at the N-10 position and is a potent inhibitor of dihydrofolate reductase. It has better cellular uptake and polyglutamation and greater preclinical antitumour activity than methotrexate. An early phase II trial had a promising response rate of 32% in 20 previously treated patients[41] but, as so often happens, the response rate has fallen as larger trials have been performed.[42] *Trimetrexate* is a new lipophilic antifolate that differs from classic antifolates in that it is not polyglutamated but enters cells by a different mechanism and accumulates to give higher intracellular concentrations. The maximum tolerated dose varies widely among patients, depending on several factors, including serum albumin concentration, schedule, and presence or absence of hepatic metastases.[43] As a single agent it has only modest activity in non-small cell lung cancer.[44] Preclinical studies, however, suggest that it may act synergistically with 5-fluorouracil and this combination may be worth evaluating.

The pyrimidine antimetabolite *gemcitabine* (difluorodeoxycytidine) is an analogue of cytosine arabinoside (Ara-c) and has preclinical activity in several murine and human tumour cell lines (including those resistant to Ara-c) and in lung xenografts. The side effects are schedule dependent fever and hypotension. It has moderate activity in non-small cell lung cancer, with a 24% partial response rate in 29 evaluable patients who had not previously had any treatment.[45]

Of three new alkylating agents that have been assessed, two have modest activity. *Fotemustine* is a chloronitrosourea that alkylates and carbamoylates DNA. An overall response rate of 21% was found in 29 evaluable patients, 24 of whom had had previous treatment.[46] A subsequent study, using a different schedule, resulted in a poorer response rate.[47] TCNU—(1-(2-chloroethyl)-3-2 (dimethylaminosulfonyl)-ethyl-1-nitrosourea)—is a water soluble nitrosourea, which given orally is reported to have a 14% response rate as a single agent in previously untreated patients.[48]

Studies on biological response modifiers are disappointing in non-small cell lung cancer. An objective response rate of 4% was achieved in 73 evaluable patients with metastatic non-small cell lung cancer who had been randomised to receive interleukin-2 (30×10^6 U/m^2) or interleukin-2 plus interferon-β (6×10^6 U/m^2) intravenously three times a week. There was no significant difference between the two groups, though the overall median survival of 35·6 weeks was longer than that seen in historical controls.[49] In a small trial of 12 evaluable patients a 33% response rate was achieved with the combination of interleukin-2 and tumour necrosis factor α.[50]

New targets and future directions for the treatment of lung cancer

New targets for treatment will, it is hoped, come from an increased understanding of the biology of tumour growth control and metastasis. Several approaches are possible.

Autocrine growth control

Lung cancer, and in particular small cell lung cancer, is associated with the production of a series of autocrine growth factors that stimulate malignant cell proliferation. These include bombesin like peptides, such as the mammalian homologue of bombesin, gastrin releasing peptide, insulin like growth factor I and transferrin (see chapter 4).[51] It has been shown, for example, that insulin like growth factor I is an autocrine growth factor in human small cell lung cancer and that in vitro tumour cell growth can be inhibited by monoclonal antibodies against insulin like growth factor I and its major receptor.[52] This raises the possibility of using antibodies or oligopeptide analogue drugs directed against the receptor. Gastrin releasing peptide has also been shown to be an important growth factor for human small cell lung cancer.[53] We are currently investigating a group of 11-amino acid oligopeptide analogues of substance P, a sensory neurotransmitter, and looking at the effects on the growth of human small cell lung cancer xenografts. Some of these analogues are powerful inhibitors of human lung cancer growth in vitro and they are thought to act at least in part through inhibition of gastrin releasing peptide. Preliminary studies also show activity in xenografts,[54] and have opened the way for early clinical trials.

Molecular genetics

Lung cancer is associated with activation of dominant proto-oncogenes or inactivation of recessive tumour suppressor genes.[55] Overexpression of the *myc* family of proto-oncogenes results in increased proliferation of human lung cell cancer cell lines[56] and could be a target for therapeutic intervention. For example, Phorbol esters, which have the ability to inhibit c-*myc* transcription, can be used to slow growth of leukaemic cells. The most common cytogenetic abnormality seen in lung cancer is a 3p deletion, principally in the 14–23 region.[57] This may represent loss of one or more recessive oncogenes, resulting in permissive expression of the malignant phenotype. Although the molecular consequences of this are not yet understood, a number of genes mapped to 3p are being investigated as potential candidates. Mutations in genes of other chromosomes, notably 13q (retinoblastoma), 17p (p53), and 11p (Wilms' tumour related gene) are common in lung cancer and would also be targets for future treatment. Exploitation of these advances is certainly a challenge and the subject of much "venture" capital investment. This is particularly true in the case of antisense olgonucleotides. These are short, synthetic, single strand nucleotides containing sequences complementary to the target nucleic acid. By virtue of the highly specific sequences of antisense oligonucleotides, it is hoped they could usefully block expression of defined oncogenes. Successful inhibition of c-*myc* expression with subsequent reduction in cell proliferation has already been achieved in vitro in this way.[58] There are many practical difficulties to be overcome with this approach in vivo; these include nuclease degradation of synthetic oligonucleotides and difficulties of cellular access.

Haematopoietic growth factors

The dose and frequency of cytotoxic drugs are often limited by myelosuppression. Use of the haematopoietic growth factors (colony stimulating factors, or CSFs) help the recovery rate of progenitor cells within the bone marrow after chemotherapy, resulting in earlier resolution of neutropenia (see chapter 8).[59]

Neutrophil recovery can be accelerated in a dose and schedule dependent manner with granulocyte CSF or granulocyte-macrophage CSF.[60] The potential benefits of CSFs for patients with lung cancer are currently under investigation. It is hoped that a survival advantage is achieved by avoiding dose reductions and delays or by permitting dose escalation or intensification.[61] CSFs, however, are ineffective in ameliorating drug induced thrombocytopenia commonly seen after carboplatin treatment, for example. Agents such as interleukin-I, which act on early multipotent progenitors, are currently under investigation.[62]

Improving quality of life

Despite its limited impact on survival, cytotoxic chemotherapy has a useful role in symptom relief[63] and may be cost effective when analysed by quality adjusted survival.[64] Development of cytotoxic drug analogues with better side effect profiles has an important part to play in improving quality of life. Clear benefits have been achieved in the management of emesis resulting from chemotherapy with $5HT_3$ antagonists, and continued research efforts to improve quality of life must be encouraged.[64] Cachexia is often a distressing symptom in patients with cancer and attempts have been made to use drugs to improve nutrition. *Medroxyprogesterone acetate* has been evaluated by a double blind, randomised, placebo controlled trial in patients with advanced cancer. The patients receiving medroxyprogesterone acetate had a significant improvement in appetite and in indicators of nutrition.[65] In a similarly designed trial patients with unresectable non-small cell lung cancer receiving hydrazine sulphate had a higher energy intake and serum albumin concentration than the placebo group.[66]

Conclusion

Prospects for conventional treatment of lung cancer remain poor. Our increasing understanding of the biology of the disease will help to identify new molecular targets for which effective drugs can be designed. Clinical trials should allow new drugs to be tested prudently early in the course of the disease, but at the same time give the patient the best chance of a good quality of life and prolonged survival.

1 Office of Population Census and Surveys. *Cancer Statistics: Registrations, England & Wales 1983*. London: HMSO, 1986.

2 Souhami R, Law K. Longevity in small cell lung cancer. A report to the Lung Cancer Subcommittee of the United Kingdom Coordinating Committee for Cancer Research. *Br J Cancer* 1990;**61**:584–9.

3 Splinter TAW. Chemotherapy in advanced non-small cell lung cancer. *Eur J Cancer* 1990;**26**:1093–9.

4 Carney DN. Biology of small cell lung cancer. *Lancet* 1992;**339**:843–6.

5 Joss RA, Cavalli F, Goldhirsch A, *et al*. New drugs in small cell lung cancer. *Cancer Treat Rev* 1986;**13**:157–76.

6 Clark P, Talbot D, Price C, *et al*. Single agent etoposide in untreated extensive small cell lung cancer [abstract]. *Lung Cancer* 1988;**4**:108.

7 Issell BF, Einhorn LH, Comis RL, *et al*. Multicenter phase II trial of etoposide in refractory small cell lung cancer. *Cancer Treat Rev* 1985;**69**:127–8.

8 Bork E, Hansen M, Dombernowsky P, *et al*. Teniposide (VM-26), an overlooked highly active agent in SCLC: results of a phase II trial in untreated patients. *J Clin Oncol* 1986;**4**:524–7.

9 Creech RH, Tritcher D, Ettinger DS, *et al*. Phase II study of PALA, amsacrine, teniposide and zinostatin in small cell lung cancer (EDT 2579). *Cancer Treat Rep* 1984;**68**:1183–4.

10 Smith IE, Harland SJ, Robinson BD, *et al*. Carboplatin: a very active new cisplatin analogue of small cell lung cancer. *Cancer Treat Rep* 1985;**69**:43–6.

11 Cullen MH, Smith SR, Benfield GFA, Woodruffe CM. Testing new drugs in untreated small cell lung cancer may prejudice the results of standard practice: a phase II study of oral idarubicin in extensive disease. *Cancer Treat Rep* 1987;**71**:1227–30.

12 Lund B, Hansen F, Hansen M, *et al*. Phase II study of 1,2,4-triglycidylurazol (TGU) in previously untreated and treated patients with small cell lung cancer. *Eur J Cancer Clin Oncol* 1987;**23**:1031–3.

13 Malik STA, Rayner H, Fletcher J, *et al*. Phase II trial of mitozantrone as first-line chemotherapy for extensive small cell lung cancer. *Cancer Treat Rep* 1987;**71**:1291–2.

14 Jackson D, Cruz J, White D, *et al*. Cisplatin in extensive small cell lung cancer: a randomised trial by the Piedmont Oncology Association. *Proc Am Soc Clin Oncol* 1989;**8**:222.

15 Cohen EA, Gralla RJ, Kris MG, *et al*. Phase II studies in small cell lung cancer: an analysis of 97 trials. *Proc Am Soc Clin Oncol* 1985;**4**:1190.

16 Grant SC, Gralla RJ, Kris MG, *et al*. Single agent chemotherapy trials in small cell lung cancer 1970 to 1990: The case for studies in previously treated patients. *J Clin Oncol* 1992;**10**:484–98.

17 Ettinger DS. Evaluation of new drugs in untreated patients with small cell lung cancer: its time has come. *J Clin Oncol* 1990;**8**:374–7.

18 Moore TD, Korn EL. Phase II trial design considerations for small cell lung cancer. *JNCI* 1992;**84**:150–4.

19 Gottlieb JA, Luce JK. Treatment of malignant melanoma with camptothecin (NSC-100880). *Cancer Chemother Rep* 1972;**56**:103–6.

20 Ohno R, Okada K, Masoaka T, *et al*. An early phase II study of CPT-11: a new derivative of camptothecin for the treatment of leukaemia and lymphoma. *J Clin Oncol* 1990;**8**:1907–12.

21 Negoro S, Fukuoka M, Niitani H, *et al*. Phase II study of CPT-11, a new camptothecin derivative in small cell lung cancer. *Proc Am Soc Clin Oncol* 1991;**10**:241.

22 Chabot GG, Barilero I, Armand JP, *et al*. Pharmacokinetics of the camptothecin analogue CPT-11 and its active metabolite SN38 in cancer patients. *Proc Am Assoc Cancer Res* 1991;**32**:175.

23 Blackstein M, Eisenhauer EA, Wierzbicki R, Yoshida S. Epirubicin in extensive small cell lung cancer: a phase II study in previously untreated patients: a National Cancer Institute of Canada Clinical Trials Group Study. *J Clin Oncol* 1990;**8**:385–9.

24 Eckhardt S, Kolaric K, Vukas D, *et al*. Phase II study of 4'-epi-doxorubicin in patients with untreated extensive small cell lung cancer. South-Eastern European Oncology Group. *Med Oncol Tumor Pharmacother* 1990;**7**:19–23.

25 Montalar J, Rosell R, Aparicio, J. Phase II trial of pirarubicin in previously treated small cell lung cancer (SCLC) patients. *Ann Oncol* 1992;**3**(Suppl 5):38.

26 Slevin ML, Clark PI, Joel SP, *et al*. A randomised trial to evaluate the effect of schedule on the activity of etoposide in small cell lung cancer. *J Clin Oncol* 1989;**7**:1333–40.

27 Einhorn LH, Pennington K, McClean J. Phase II trial of daily oral VP16 in refractory small cell lung cancer: a Hoosier Oncology Group Study. *Semin Oncol* 1990;**17**(Suppl 1):32–5.

28 Bork E, Sigsgaard T, Nissen KM, *et al.* Etoposide and Teniposide in untreated small cell lung cancer (SCLC). *Lung Cancer* 1991;7(Suppl):121.
29 Leteurtre F, Madalengoitia J, Orr A, *et al.* Rational design and molecular effects of a new topoisomerase II inhibitor, Azatoxin. *Cancer Res* 1992;52:4478–83.
30 Einhorn LH. Ifosfamide in small cell lung cancer. *Semin Oncol* 1989;16(Suppl 3):19–21.
31 Cantwell BMJ, Bozzini JM, Corris P, *et al.* Ifosfamide after VP16, doxorubicin and vincristine for small cell lung cancer. *Eur J Cancer Clin Oncol* 1988;24:123–9.
32 Loehrer PJ, Birch R, Kramer BS, *et al.* Ifosfamide in the treatment of small cell lung cancer and non-small cell lung cancer. An SECSG Trial. *Cancer Treat Rep* 1986;1:919–20.
33 Thatcher N, Lind M, De Campos E, *et al.* Novel approaches with ifosfamide in small cell lung cancer. *Semin Oncol* 1992;19(suppl 1):68–77.
34 Thatcher N, Lind M. Carboplatin in small cell lung cancer. *Semin Oncol* 1990;17(suppl 2):40–8.
35 Clamon G, Ozer H, Herndon M, Perry Scalzo A, Green MR. Activity of interleukin-2 (IL-2) in patients (pts) with extensive small cell lung cancer. *Proc Am Soc Clin Oncol* 1992;11:312.
36 Mattson K, Niiranen A, Holsti LR, *et al.* Natural alpha interferon as maintenance therapy for small cell lung cancer. *Lung Cancer* 1991;7(suppl):127.
37 Jett JR, Su JQ, Maksymiuk AW. Phase III trial of recombinant interferon-γ (rIFN-γ) in complete responders (CR) with small cell lung cancer SCC). *Proc Am Soc Clin Oncol* 1992;11:287.
38 Asakawa M, Fujita A, Fukuoka M, *et al.* Phase II study of CPT-11, new camptothecin derivative, in previously untreated non-small cell lung cancer (NSCLC). *Lung Cancer* 1991;7(Suppl):125.
39 Yokoyama A, Furuse K, Niitani H, *et al.* Multi-institutional phase II study of navelbine (vinorelbine) in non-small cell lung cancer. *Proc Am Soc Clin Oncol* 1992;11:287.
40 Jones AL, Davies C, Smith IE. Phase II study of zeniplatin, an active new agent in advanced non-small cell lung cancer (NSCLC). *Lung Cancer* 1991;7(Suppl):125.
41 Shum KY, Kris MG, Gralla RJ, Burke MT, Marks LD, Heelan RT. Phase II study of 1-ethyl-10-deaza-aminopterin in patients with stage III and IV non-small cell lung cancer. *J Clin Oncol* 1988;6:446–50.
42 Soulhami R, Hartley J, Allen R, Rudd R, Harper P, Spiro S. Phase II study of 10-Edam (10-ethyl-10-deaza-aminopterin) in untreated advanced non-small cell lung cancer. *Proc Am Soc Clin Oncol* 1991;10:252.
43 Bertino JR, Lin JT, Chasmore AR, *et al.* Clinical pharmacology and metabolism of trimetrexate. *Semin Oncol* 1988;15:8–9.
44 Gesme DH, Su JQ, Jett JR. Randomized phase II trial with amonafide (AMF) or trimetrexate (TMTX) for stage IV non-small cell lung cancer (NSCLC). *Proc Am Soc Clin Oncol* 1992;11:310.
45 Anderson H, Lund B, Hansen HH, Walling J, Thatcher N. Gemcitabine in non-small cell lung cancer. *Proc Am Soc Clin Oncol* 1991;10:247.
46 Monnier A, Pujol JL, Cerrina ML, *et al.* Fotemustine in non-small cell lung cancer: phase II study in 32 patients with poor prognostic factors. *Proc Am Soc Clin Oncol* 1991;10:248.
47 Le Cesne A, Le Chevalier T, Marty M, *et al.* A new administration schedule of Fotemustine in non small cell lung cancer (NSCLC): final results of a phase III study with a D1-2-3 schedule. *Ann Oncol* 1992;3(Suppl 5):35.
48 Sorensen JM, Bach F, Dombernowski P, Vibe-Petersen J, Hansen JJ. TCNU in adenocarcinoma of the lung: a phase II study with divided doses. *Ann Oncol* 1990;1:299–300.
49 Krigel R, Lynch E, Kucuk O, *et al.* Interleukin-2 (IL-2) therapies prolong survival in metastatic non-small cell lung cancer. *Proc Am Soc Clin Oncol* 1991;10:246.
50 Yang SC, Owen-Schaub L, Mendiguren-Rodriguez A, Grimm EA, Hong WK, Roth JA. Combination immunotherapy for non-small cell lung cancer. Results with interleukin-2 and tumour necrosis factor-a. *J Thorac Cardiovasc Surg* 1990;99:8–12.
51 Woll PJ. Growth factors and lung cancer. *Thorax* 1991;46:924–9.
52 Macauley VM, Everard MJ, Teale JD, *et al.* Autocrine function for insulin-like growth factor I in human small cell lung cancer cell lines and fresh tumour cells. *Cancer Res* 1990;50:2511–7.
53 Cuttitta F, Carney DN, Mulshine J, *et al.* Bombesin-like peptides can function as autocrine growth factors in human small cell lung cancer. *Nature* 1985;316:823–6.
54 Langdon S, Sethi T, Ritchie A, *et al.* Broad spectrum neuropeptide antagonists inhibit the growth of small cell lung cancer in vivo. *Cancer Res* 1992;52:4554–7.

55 Minna J, Maneckjee R, D'Amico D, et al. Mutations in dominant and recessive oncogenes, and the expression of opioid and nicotine receptors in the pathogenesis of lung cancer. *Proc Am Assoc Cancer Res* 1991;**32**:445–6.

56 Johnson BE, Ihde DC, Makuch RW, et al. Myc family oncogene amplification in tumour cell lines established from small cell lung cancer patients and its relationship to clinical status and course. *J Clin Invest* 1987;**79**:1629–34.

57 Kok K, Osinger J, Carritt B, et al. Deletion of a DNA sequence at the chromosomal region 3p21 in all major types of lung cancer. *Nature* 1987;**330**:578–81.

58 Wickstrom EL, Bacon JA, Gonzalez A, et al. Human promyelocytic leukaemic HL-60 cell proliferation and c-myc protein expression are inhibited by an antisense pentadeca neucleotide targetted against c-myc mRNA. *Proc Natl Acad Sci USA* 1988;**85**:1028–32.

59 Thatcher N. Haematopoietic growth factors and lung cancer. *Thorax* 1992;**47**:119–26.

60 Metcalf D. The colony stimulating factors, discovery, development and clinical applications. *Cancer* 1990;**65**:2185–206.

61 Drings P, Fischer JR. Biology and clinical use of GMCSF in lung cancer. *Lung* 1990;**168**(Suppl): 1059–68.

62 Tepler I, Elias A, Young D, et al. Use of recombinant human interleukin-3 (IL3) after "ICE" chemotherapy for non-small cell lung cancer (NSCLC); effect on haematological recovery. *Proc Am Soc Clin Oncol* 1992;**11**:296.

63 Hardy JR, Noble T, Smith IE. Symptom relief with moderate dose chemotherapy (mitomycin C, vinblastine, ciplatin) in advanced non-small cell lung cancer. *Br J Cancer* 1989;**60**:764–6.

64 Rosenthal MA, Webster PJ, Gebski RC, et al. The cost of small cell lung cancer. *Lung Cancer* 1991;**7**(Suppl):145.

65 Talbot DC, Joel SP, Stubbs L, et al. A randomised, double blind, placebo controlled trial of medroxyprogesterone acetate (MPA) in cancer cachexia. *Br J Cancer* 1988;**58**:267.

66 Chlebowski RT, Bulcavage L, Grosvenor M, et al. Hydrazine sulfate influence on nutritional status and survival in non-small cell lung cancer. *J Clin Oncol* 1990;**8**:9–15.

67 Manegold C, Loechner S, Bachmann P, Burk K, Drings P. Oral ifosamide in elderly and/or unfit patients with small cell lung cancer (SCLC)—A Phase II study. *Ann Oncol* 1992;**3**(Suppl 5):38.

68 Ettinger D, Finkelstein D, Ritch P, Bonomi P, Blum R. Randomized trial of single agents vs combination chemotherapy in extensive stage small cell lung cancer (SCLC). *Proc Am Soc Clin Oncol* 1992;**11**:295.

69 Giaccone G, Donadio M, Bonardi G, et al. Teniposide in the treatment of small cell lung cancer: The influence of prior chemotherapy. *J Clin Oncol* 1988;**6**:1264–70.

70 Harding M, Docherty V, Mackie R, Dorward A, Kaye S. Phase II studies of mitoxolomide in melanoma, lung and ovarian cancer. *Eur J Cancer Clin Oncol* 1989;**25**:785–8.

71 Jassem J, Karnicka-Modkowska H, van Pottelsberghe C, et al. EORTC Phase II study of navelbine (NVB) in previously treated patients (PTS) with small cell lung carcinoma (SCLC). *Proc Am Soc Clin Oncol* 1992;**11**:309.

72 Ettinger DS, Finkelstein DM, Abeloff MD, Bonomi PD. Justification for evaluating new anticancer drugs in selected untreated patients with a chemotherapy-sensitive advanced cancer: an ECOG randomised study. *Proc Am Soc Clin Oncol* 1990;**9**:224.

73 Abratt R, Bezwoda W, Falkson G, et al. Efficacy and safety of gemcitabine in non-small cell lung cancer. Phase II study results. *Ann Oncol* 1992;**3**(Suppl 5):28.

74 Lund B, Ryberg M, Meidal P, et al. A phase II study of gemcitabine in non-small cell lung cancer (NSCLC) using a twice weekly schedule. *Ann Oncol* 1992;**3**(Suppl 5):31.

75 Chang A, Kim K, Glick J, et al. Phase II trial of taxol in patients with stage IV non-small cell lung cancer (NSCLC). *Proc Am Soc Clin Oncol* 1992;**11**:293.

76 Gatzemeier U, Heckmayr M, Hossfeld DK, Zschaber R, Achterrath W, Lenaz L. Phase II study of carboplatin in untreated, inoperable non-small cell lung cancer. *Cancer Chemother Pharmacol* 1990;**26**:369–72.

77 Feld R, Wierzbicki R, Walde D, et al. A phase II trial of high dose epirubicin in patients with untreated extensive non-small cell lung cancer. *Proc Am Soc Clin Oncol* 1990;**2**:240.

78 Maroun J. Clinical response to trimetrexate as sole therapy for non-small cell lung cancer. *Semin Oncol* 1988;**15**(Suppl 2):17–21.

79 Giaccone G, Donadio M, Ferrati P, et al. Teniposide in the treatment of non-small cell lung carcinoma. *Cancer Treat Rep* 1987;**71**:83–5.

80 Fukuda M, Shinkai I, Eguchi K, *et al*. Phase II study of (glycolate-0·0′) diammineplatinum (II), a novel platinum complex in the treatment of non-small cell lung cancer. *Cancer Chemother Pharmacol* 1990;**26**:393–6.
81 Drings P, Gunther IU, Gatzemeier U, *et al*. Pirarubicin in advanced non-small cell lung cancer. A trial of the phase I/II study group of the Association for Medical Oncology of the German Cancer Society. *Onkologie* 1990;**13**:180–4.
82 Eberhardt W, Weidmann B, Niederle N, *et al*. Iododoxorubicin in advanced non-small cell lung cancer (NSCLC)—A phase II study. *Ann Oncol* 1992;**3**(Suppl 5):29.
83 Rose C, Lad TE, Kilton LJ, *et al*. Phase II trial of 4′deoxydoxorubicin for unresectable non-small cell bronchogenic carcinoma. An Illinois Cancer Council study. *Invest New Drugs* 1990;**8**:97–9.
84 Kokron O, Maca S, De Gregorio M, Ciottoli GB. Phase II study of lonidamine in non-small cell lung cancer: final report. *Br J Cancer* 1990;**61**:316–8.

10 Quality of life

PENELOPE HOPWOOD, ANN CULL

The majority of patients with lung cancer are treated with palliative intent, and traditionally, outcome has been measured in terms of the extent and duration of tumour response and patients' survival. In the past decade differences between treatments, as measured by these biological indices, have been small and it has become increasingly relevant to individual patient care and to policy making to compare the cost, in both human and economic terms, at which any such gain is achieved. To this end the range of psychosocial effects caused by lung cancer and its treatment has been comprehensively reviewed.[1 2]

Scales for monitoring toxicity related to treatment and performance status are still widely used but are inadequate to assess key aspects of patients' experience, such as pain, fatigue, and nausea, which are essentially subjective. Furthermore, clinicians recognise that patients with apparently similar toxicity or performance status ratings may experience substantially different quality of life when this is more globally assessed.

The concept of quality of life is generally accepted as a basis for clinical decision making, but its assessment in routine practice has historically been a matter of clinical judgment. It is therefore unsystematic and open to bias. More reproducible methods of quality of life assessment are now required for use in: (i) auditing clinical practice; (ii) evaluating treatment outcome in clinical trials; (iii) informed decision making in the care of individual patients; (iv) justifying needs for supportive services; and (v) allocating resources for medical services. Most progress has been made in the second of these quality of life outcomes of clinical trials, which will be the focus for this chapter.

161

Definition of quality of life

Clinicians frequently express the concern that quality of life is a subjective concept varying from individual to individual and therefore impossible to define or measure scientifically. It is generally agreed that health related quality of life is a multidimensional construct concerned with the impact of physical symptoms of the disease and treatment related side effects on patients' functioning and psychosocial wellbeing. Specific research questions may justify a narrower focus, but studies sampling only one of these domains cannot adequately reflect patients' global quality of life. A second point of consensus is that wherever possible, emphasis should be placed on the subjective experience of the person whose quality of life is in question. Hence attention has focused particularly on the development of questionnaires completed by patients themselves.

Quality of life components

- Impact of disease symptoms
- Side effects of treatment
- Ability to function
- Psychosocial wellbeing

Quality of life assessment methods for lung cancer

It follows from this definition that indirect indicators such as time spent in hospital or days off work may provide valuable information for evaluating the socioeconomic outcome of treatments, but on their own they are inadequate measures of quality of life.

In designing a protocol for a quality of life study it is crucial to begin with a clearly defined research question so that selection of the appropriate assessment strategy and relevant instruments follows logically. Measures designed to detect group differences in treatment response will not provide adequate information for clinical decision making for individual patients, and there is no all-purpose "gold standard" measure of quality of life. Much dissatisfaction expressed about quality of life assessment stems from unrealistic expectations of what can be achieved.

A bewildering array of approaches has emerged to assess quality of life end points, ranging from generic health outcome measures to instruments designed specifically for use with patients with cancer. Generic measures such as the Sickness Impact Profile[3] or Medical Outcome Study (MOS) Short Form General Health Survey[4] were designed for use across a wide range of chronic diseases. They allow outcomes to be compared across patient populations, which may be necessary for cost effectiveness studies but they are often unsuitable for assessing the symptoms and side-effects of interventions in specific patient groups.

On the other hand, more specific measures are intended to be responsive to disease and treatment related changes affecting quality of life, but they may fail to provide sufficiently comprehensive data for comparison with other patient populations.

The range of questionnaires developed specifically for patients with cancer, together with guidelines for selecting appropriate measures, have been described elsewhere and there are some excellent texts available.[5-7] In particular, a review by Cella and Tulsky[8] gives an up to date appraisal of 24 quality of life scales, many of which are published in an Appendix.[9] An updated version of the *Quality of life bibliography and indexes* (compiled by Burroughs Wellcome) has been published[10]: relevant publications are indexed by instrument and by therapeutic category.

The first developed measures, Linear (or Visual) Analogue Self-Assessment Scales (LASA or VASA) have frequently been used with cancer patients. They are purported to be sensitive to small changes, but one study directly compared a LASA scale with a categorical response scale and failed to demonstrate differential sensitivity.[11] Others, however, found that LASA scores correlated well with performance and reflected morbidity related to treatment.[12] The LASA format may also be more difficult for patients to understand and complete and these scales are time consuming to score.

The Functional Living Index–Cancer (FLIC)[13] has also been widely used with cancer patients, initially designed on the analogue format, but now including a seven point scale. Reservation about the suitability of the FLIC for use with patients with lung cancer has arisen from a comparative trial of supportive care and combination chemotherapy in non-small cell lung cancer[14] in which the FLIC was found to provide insufficient data about functional problems and to be insensitive to clinically important change.

Clearly, more comprehensive information is required to assess adequately the quality of life of patients with lung cancer.

Generic and specific requirements can be reconciled by the adoption of a modular approach whereby a "core" instrument covers a range of issues relevant to a broad spectrum of cancer patients and is supplemented by more specific subscales or "modules" to assess aspects of quality of life of particular importance to specific subgroups. This strategy promoted by the EORTC Study Group on Quality of Life[15] has been taken up by others and additional items for patients with lung cancer are being developed for use not only with the EORTC's Core Quality of Life Measure (QLQ-C30)[16] but also with the Rotterdam Symptom Checklist (RSCL)[17] and with the new Functional Assessment of Cancer Therapy (FACT) Scale.[18]

EORTC QLQ-C30 and lung cancer module

The EORTC Quality of Life Study Group has developed a 30 item self-report quality of life questionnaire (QLQ-C30) for use in cancer clinical trials. Recently reported results of the second field study[16] confirmed the QLQ-C30 as reliable and valid for use in multicultural clinical research to assess the physical, psychological, and social functioning, symptom levels, and global quality of life of patients with cancer. The instrument is responsive to clinical change and has proved acceptable to patients. A substantial data set is now accruing from its increasing use worldwide by members of the Quality of Life Group.

In two field studies involving more than 800 patients with lung cancer the Group collected specific data using an additional 13 item subscale (the Lung Cancer Module). This covers disease symptoms such as pain, dyspnoea, cough, and side-effects of treatment such as dysphagia, hair loss, and neuropathy. Although the module showed satisfactory reliability and responsiveness to clinical change, some improvements have been proposed[19] and the revised version will require further field testing before being made available for general use.

Rotterdam Symptom Checklist (RSCL)

The RSCL is a 30 item checklist designed for use with cancer patients. It covers physical and psychological wellbeing and includes eight items to assess activities of daily living plus one item for global quality of life. It has been used in studies of small cell lung cancer[20][21] and has been recommended by a working group of the MRC Cancer Therapy Committee reporting on Quality of Life instruments.[22] It can be used in conjunction with the Hospital Anxiety and Depression Scale (HADS).[23] As a result of the Cancer Therapy Committee recommendations, the MRC Lung Cancer Working Party has now included this combination of instruments in its clinical trials. Items have been added to the original RSCL to cover lung cancer symptoms and specific treatment effects, and work is underway at the MRC cancer trials office to examine the factor structure of the checklist, with particular interest in the physical items and lung cancer specific symptoms.

Hospital Anxiety and Depression Scale (HADS)

This 14 item scale was designed for use with medical outpatients to measure psychological distress. It has two subscales—depression and anxiety—each of seven items and is quick and easy to complete and score. It has been extensively used in a variety of medical settings, but especially in oncology. The authors have recommended threshold scores which enable the questionnaire to screen for clinical levels of depression and anxiety.

Assessment of quality of life

- LASA (VASA)
- FLIC
- QLQ-C30
- RSCL
- FACT
- HADS
- PDC

Patient diary card (PDC)

The need to provide clinicians with detailed information about change in a limited number of symptoms was instrumental in the development of a patient diary card by the MRC Lung Cancer Working Party.[24] This contained a few simple questions about mood, anxiety, overall condition, activity, major symptoms and nausea and vomiting.

The diary card yields reliable, repeatable data[25][26] and is sensitive to changes provoked by different chemotherapy and radiotherapy regimens in patients with small cell and non-small cell lung cancer. Its disadvantages are its limited coverage and disappointing compliance.

Functional Assessment of Cancer Therapy Scale (FACT)

This 33 item general cancer quality of life measure has been carefully developed over the past five years by an American team,[18] according to sound principles of test construction. Patients with lung cancer were represented in the validation process of this instrument which produces five subscale scores for physical, functional, social and emotional wellbeing and satisfaction with the treatment relationship. Uniquely this measure includes a patient rated appraisal, on a 0 to 10 scale, of the effect each dimension has on overall quality of life, thereby increasing the measure's potential usefulness in cost-effectiveness studies. The general scale has fewer physical items than many cancer specific measures and the authors report its applicability, with minor modification, to other chronic disease groups. Disease specific issues can then be appended as a sixth subscale of "additional concerns".

Nine items are proposed for lung cancer, covering symptoms such as weight loss and dyspnoea and including an item on regret about smoking. There is an additional rating of the extent to which these concerns affect patients' quality of life. More published data are required about the performance of this promising general instrument and the lung cancer specific scale before its use can be recommended.

An important consideration in selecting a quality of life measure is the extent to which it meets acceptable standards of reliability, validity, and sensitivity to change over time.[27] The psychometric properties of an instrument cannot be assumed to hold across patient populations that differ in disease type or functional status. Results should always be interpreted with these limitations in mind.

Cost effectiveness

The role of economic factors in cancer care has become increasingly important, alongside considerations of effectiveness,[28] and the use of quality of life measures for allocating limited resources has proved controversial. It is important to distinguish between an economic evaluation using a cost effectiveness technique, which expresses the additional cost of each additional unit of benefit for one treatment over another, from a cost utility analysis, where the benefits are expressed in terms of survival adjusted for quality. This quality adjustment uses "utilities" to compare, numerically, the value of a given health state to a perfect (or usual) health state, on the assumption that reduced quality is equivalent to reduced duration in perfect health. This may not, of course, reflect patient preferences which may in any case vary widely.

To date, there have been few published economic evaluations of lung cancer treatment,[29] or indeed of cancer treatment in general, although oncology departments have been urged to consider cost aspects of cancer care.[30 31]

Some interesting methodological approaches combining quality and quantity of life data have been published,[32] but developmental work is required before these can be generally accepted and applied to clinical trials. There is still a strong lobby in favour of retaining multidimensional end points to assess treatment outcomes,[33] while the cost effectiveness approach serves a different (socioeconomic) purpose—that is, to evaluate health states across diseases and inform decision making in resource allocation.

Achievements so far

The number of published lung cancer clinical trials in which quality of life has been assessed remains disappointingly small, but a considerable amount of research is now underway. A detailed review of work to date cannot be encompassed here, but major areas will be highlighted.

"Proxy" quality of life assessments

The need to include quality end points has led to the publication of studies in which outcome measures purporting to reflect quality of life have fallen short of the definition given here. The evaluation of performance and other basic clinical variables, such as body weight, respiratory scores, global toxicity and patient dropout rates, have all been used and reported under the rubric "Quality of Life".[34-38] At best they can be regarded as only "proxy" measures of the impact of treatment, because they are not completed by

167

patients themselves and provide limited information. Moreover, concern has been voiced that performance status is an unreliable measure of patients' wellbeing. Although some groups have reported good correlation between Karnofsky Performance (KP) scores and other quality of life measures,[13 39] others have not. For example, Geddes et al[26] found Karnofsky scores insensitive to change in patients with small cell lung cancer in whom worsening treatment toxicity was identified by a daily diary card, and Fernandez[36] found no correlation between Karnofsky scores and patient generated symptoms ratings (measured by VASA scales) in predicting response to treatment.

Quality of life studies in non-small cell lung cancer

Only a small proportion of patients with non-small cell lung cancer are entered into clinical trials, very few of which have reported quality of life outcomes. It is, however, relevant to reflect on the Canadian findings that most specialists who treat lung cancer, when presented with the hypothetical scenario of non-small cell lung cancer themselves, would not consent to participate as subjects in a range of clinical trials drawn from contemporary practice.[40]

The lack of interesting research questions regarding treatment approaches and failure to improve survival in these patients have also contributed to a sense of pessimism in this area. For a very large number of patients with metastatic non-small cell lung cancer, an improvement in chemotherapy may be the only realistic possibility of increasing survival, but few active agents have been identified. And the use of chemotherapy is controversial because of low response rates in the face of moderate toxicity, and so the cost:benefit ratio is crucial to an evaluation of outcome.

Regrettably, most studies assessing quality of life during treatment for non-small cell lung cancer have relied on "proxy" measures. It is not surprising that this approach has led to contradictory findings when used in heterogeneous groups of patients undergoing a variety of treatment regimens.

In a randomised comparative trial of chemotherapy and radiotherapy using a patient rated psychosocial scale, the results of a Norwegian quality of life study[41] suggested that patients were willing to trade treatment toxicity for the chance of responding to treatment. Patients' wellbeing scores correlated closely with symptoms related to disease but poorly with adverse treatment effects.

Little is known about the impact of palliative radiotherapy on patients' quality of life. In patients who respond poorly, attempts have been made to simplify palliative treatments. Thus the symptom relief achieved with different policies of thoracic radiotherapy was compared in two randomised multicentre trials conducted by the MRC Lung Cancer Working Party. In the first of these, a standard 30 Gy in 10 fractions regimen was compared with a 17 Gy in two fractions[42]; subsequently, the two fraction regimen was compared with a single fraction of 10 Gy.[43] Patients reported symptoms using the MRC Daily Diary Card during their first six months in the trial. This evaluation was limited to a simple range of symptoms but represents an important step in trying to assess quality of life in a multicentre, clinical setting. Results in terms of adverse effects and palliation were similar for the 10 compared with the two fraction treatments. In the second trial, however, although clinicians assessed palliation as broadly similar in the two fraction regimen compared with the single fraction, dysphagia was substantially greater with the two fraction regimen, as assessed by the diary card. The acceptability of the single fraction regimen was an important finding, because radiotherapists had been concerned about the potential immediate adverse effects of a large single fraction.

Considerable work is now under way to evaluate quality of life in palliative non-small cell lung cancer clinical trials, and it is hoped that the fruits of this will be apparent in the next few years.

Quality of life studies in small cell lung cancer

The MRC diary card has been the most frequently used instrument in quality of life studies in small cell lung cancer trials reported so far. Other studies have relied on psychological distress[39 44] and Simple Linear Analogues[12] to report the impact of treatment mainly in randomised trials. The EORTC scale has been used by two groups[45 46] and shown great promise, due to its rigorous field testing before release.

The MRC Patient Diary Card has been used in four small cell lung cancer trials. In the first of these[47] patients randomised to receive immediate combination chemotherapy and radiotherapy were compared with those who received these treatments selectively, as and when required, to control symptoms. Both treatment policies had their advocates in the United Kingdom, and the trial showed that using the policy of immediate treatment doubled the survival time. Quality of life assessed by the clinicians was deemed better, but adverse reactions were more common and quality of life as reported by patients was worse. Subsequently, the MRC have published the use of the diary card in a comparison of chemotherapy scheduling[48][25] in which six courses of maintenance chemotherapy were compared with no maintenance. There was no overall survival advantage with additional chemotherapy beyond six courses, though there was a suggestion that it was beneficial in patients showing a complete response to induction chemotherapy. Patients who did not receive maintenance treatment experienced a gradually deteriorating quality of life; those allocated maintenance treatment experienced additional toxicity associated with the treatment.

There is therefore no guarantee that adding quality of life end points makes the choice of treatment policy easier, but it does serve to clarify the potential trade-offs that need to be discussed with patients. Further reports are in preparation for trials comparing three and six courses of combination chemotherapy and a four drug and a two drug combination in small cell lung cancer.

In studies of palliative treatment the diary card has detected transient treatment effects that would not usually be elicited at routine clinical follow up, but compliance has been generally low, and therefore the results may not be representative. Limiting its use to patients with better performance status (KP $>70\%$) improved compliance to 68% in the study reported by Geddes et al,[26] whereas a disappointing 51% failed to return any cards at all in the MRC palliative study described above.[47] In the randomised comparative trial of four and eight cycles of chemotherapy reported by Geddes, using a diary card modelled on the MRC version, the quality of life analysis suggested that stopping chemotherapy early was associated with fewer symptoms.

A counterintuitive result was revealed by Earl et al,[49] comparing "planned" and "as required" chemotherapy in an attempt to reduce toxicity and limit the inconvenience of treatment. Survival was equivalent to the two treatment policies (despite the fact that the "as required" patients received half as much chemotherapy). Contrary to expectations, quality of life assessments in patients receiving "planned" treatment were much more favourable than the "as required" group. Such results (and there have been others in breast cancer studies) serve to highlight the potential value of quality of life research in challenging assumptions made about current treatment policies, and in particular, in questioning the view held by many that patients are "overtreated" in the palliative setting.

Compliance with the RSCL and HAD scale has been more favourable than the daily diary card in patients receiving palliative treatment. In interim analyses of an MRC clinical trial a reduction in anxiety was found during the early phase of receiving chemotherapy, although depression scores changed little.[50] An advantage of using these scales is that clinical levels of depression and anxiety can be estimated, both for individual patients and in terms of prevalence rates in study samples. An improvement in psychological wellbeing was also shown in a series of patients with small cell lung cancer randomised to receive chemotherapy by intravenous bolus or continuous pump infusion.[21] This change in wellbeing occurred in advance of any subjective improvement in physical or functional status, and the use of the infusion pump created no additional anxiety.

The results of further multicentre clinical trials using a multidimensional approach to assess the impact of treatment are awaited with interest.

Quality of life research in progress

The range of clinical areas in which quality of life evaluation is being carried out is now broad, covering many facets of lung cancer management. In patients with a poor prognosis the MRC Lung Cancer Working Party are assessing the value of early supportive treatment with or without radiotherapy in patients with non-small cell lung cancer, and of oral etoposide compared with intravenous chemotherapy in patients with small cell lung cancer. A third trial evaluating treatment policies for endobronchial obstruction for non-small cell lung cancer is now in progress and a dose intensification study is due to open for patients with small cell lung cancer and a better prognosis.

A particular area of controversy that is being researched concerns the benefits and adverse effects of prophylactic cranial irradiation (PCI) in survivors of small cell lung cancer. Conflicting evidence exists concerning the risk of cognitive impairment following PCI, and the United Kingdom Coordinating Committee on Cancer Research (UKCCCR) have recently completed a retrospective study of late central nervous system effects in 65 long term

171

survivors of small cell lung cancer. Although only a minority showed persistent abnormality on neurotoxicity grading or neurological examination, significant morbidity apparently related to treatment variables, such as initial chemotherapy and PCI dose, was detected when neuropsychometric factors were assessed (unpublished observations). A prospective randomised trial, including neuropsychometric, assessment is now in progress under the auspices of the UKCCCR to provide a more definitive answer to this controversial issue.

Quality of life and cost effectiveness are being measured in a unique United Kingdom randomised trial of non-small cell lung cancer conducted by the MRC in collaboration with the Centre for Health Economics in York, and supported by the Department of Health. Patients with inoperable non-small cell lung cancer amenable to radical radiotherapy are allocated to receive the CHART regimen (Continuous Hyperfractionated Accelerated Radiotherapy) or conventional radiotherapy. This follows promising results from a pilot study in which radiotherapy (54 Gy) was delivered in 36 fractions over 12 consecutive days.

Many individual groups within the United Kingdom are also now making quality of life an integral part of their evaluation, particularly, in studies of small cell lung cancer. The pharmaceutical industry is also increasingly interested in including these end points when introducing new anti-cancer agents in phase II and phase III trials.

Issues in implementation

Several experts have pointed out the pitfalls in implementing quality of life research[51] and clear guidelines on how to proceed are available to help the newcomer.

The most important point to address at the outset is "what is the precise question we want to answer in this trial, in terms of the impact on quality of life?" Identifying a hypothesis to test, or an expected adverse effect to assess, will enable the optimum study design and appropriate measures to be determined.

The second step is to establish that the institution or research group has the resources to support a quality of life study. This kind of work, particularly in the palliative setting, requires time and staff for data collection, and cannot always be incorporated into routine clinical activities. Yet meticulous data collection and checking are essential to avoid adding to the problems of missing data, resulting inevitably from patients who die or become too ill to complete questionnaires.

There is as yet no consensus on the best method of longitudinal analysis of quality of life data and how to deal with integral problems such as inputting missing values. Deaths from other causes, non-compliance, and patients who are lost to follow up will also have censoring effects on study data. Published guidelines for statistical methods are theoretical or, if based on trial data, often very technical.[33 52] Several groups are tackling these problems and, given its commitment to quality of life research (not only in lung cancer), the MRC Cancer Trials Office is particularly active in this area. In the meantime various approaches will be used, and the most helpful way to report such studies is to state clearly *how* the data have been analysed, specifying how missing values or cases have been dealt with. Interpretations can then be made with the knowledge of any limitations or bias.

Although some groups in the United States of America and Canada advocate the inclusion of quality of life end points in all clinical trials, it seems unrealistic to expect clinicians in the United Kingdom to endorse this, given resource limitations. Selection of trials should take account of the need for the quality of life end points to make a valid contribution to future planning of treatment and patient care.

Future directions

Several important applications for quality of life research have not yet been tackled systematically. Many clinicians have expressed a need for a very simple questionnaire for speedy use in outpatient clinics, but this may be an unrealistic request unless it is restricted to highlight limited symptoms or problem areas. Nevertheless, brief checklists are being developed[53] and justify testing to aid screening for specific problems so that more time can be spent with those in most need. Such measures could also be adapted for use in auditing clinical practice, both highlighting new areas and justifying existing areas where better support services are required.

The use of health related quality of life measures in resource allocation is another promising target, but the current state of development is limited. A central problem of using quality adjusted survival is the appropriate weighting of different health states. The necessary stages in developing QALYS (quality added life years saved) analysis have recently been described.[54] Other multistate models also warrant appraisal in trying to conceptualise life quality and quantity simultaneously.

Conclusions

The lack of a working definition for quality of life and of instruments to measure it are no longer valid excuses for failing to include quality of life end points in clinical trials. Modification of existing questionnaires and improvements in study design will continue, and clearer guidelines for data analysis will certainly be forthcoming. Where patient samples are limited, collaboration should be considered, because modest differences in quality of life may not be detected in small samples. Multidimensional end points should be retained and described in full and not aggregated into a single global score. Several centres now have expertise in this field and consultation or collaboration at the planning stage may preclude frustrating difficulties with design or analysis.

The challenge for quality of life researchers lies in those areas where its application has yet to be integrated fully. It is to be hoped that innovative treatment policies for lung cancer will also provide new stimuli in clinical trials.

1 Bernhard J, Ganz PA. Psychosocial issues in lung cancer patients: Part 1. *Chest* 1991;**99**:216–23.
2 Bernhard J, Ganz PA. Psychosocial issues in lung cancer patients: Part 2. *Chest* 1991;**99**:480–5.
3 Bergner M, Bobbitt RA, Carter WB, Gilson BS. The Sickness Impact Profile: development and final revision of a health status measure. *Med Care* 1981;**19**:787–805.
4 Stewart AL, Hays RD, Ward JE. The MOS Short Form General Health Survey: Reliability and validity in a patient population. *Med Care* 1988;**26**:724–35.
5 Osoba D, ed. *Effect of cancer on quality of life.* Boca Raton: CRC Press, 1991.
6 Spilker B, ed. *Quality of life assessments in clinical trials.* New York: Raven Press, 1990.
7 Walker SR, Rosser RM, eds. Quality of life assessment: Key issues in the 1990s. Dordrecht: Kluwer, 1993.
8 Cella DF, Tulsky DS. Measuring quality of life today: methodological aspects. *Oncology* 1990;**4**:29–38.
9 Cella DF, Tulsky DS. Quality of life measures (Appendix I). *Oncology* 1990;**4**:209–30.
10 Spilker B, Simpson RL Jnr, Tilson HH. Quality of life bibliography and indexes. 1991 update. *J Clin Res Pharm Epidemiol* 1992;**6**:205–66.
11 Guyatt GH, Townsend M, Berman L, Keller JL. A comparison of Likert and Visual Analogue Scales for measuring change in function. *J Chron Dis* 1987;**40**:1129–33.
12 Coates A, Dillenbeck CF, McNeil DR, *et al.* On the receiving end—II. Linear analogue self-assessment (LASA) in evaluation of aspects of the quality of life of cancer patients receiving therapy. *Eur J Cancer Clin Oncol* 1983;**19**:1633–7.
13 Schipper H, Clinch J, McMurray A, Levitt M. Measuring the quality of life of cancer patients. The Functional Living Index—Cancer: development and validation. *J Clin Oncol* 1984;**2**:472–83.

14 Ganz PA, Haskell CM, Figlin RA, La Soto N, Siau J. Estimating the quality of life in a clinical trial of patients with metastatic lung cancer using the Karnofsky Performance Status and the Functional Living Index—Cancer. *Cancer* 1988;**61**:849–56.

15 Aaronson NK, Bullinger M, Ahmedzai S. A modular approach to quality of life assessment in cancer clinical trials. *Rec Res Cancer Res* 1988;**111**:231–49.

16 Aaronson NK, Ahmedzai S, Bergman B, *et al*. The EORTC QLQ-C30: A quality of life instrument for use in international clinical trials in oncology. *JNCI* 1993;**85**:365–76.

17 de Haes JCJM, van Knippenberg FCE, Neijt JP. Measuring psychological and physical distress in cancer patients: structure and application of the Rotterdam Symptom Checklist. *Br J Cancer* 1990;**62**:1034–8.

18 Cella DF, Tulsky DS, Gray G, *et al*. The functional assessment of cancer therapy scale: development and validation of the general measure. *J Clin Oncol* 1993;**11**:570–9.

19 Bergman B. The EORTC QLQ Lung Cancer Module: a preliminary analysis. Internal report to the EORTC. Quality of Life Study Group. 1992.

20 Hopwood P, Thatcher T. Preliminary experience with quality of life evaluation in patients with lung cancer. *Oncology* 1990;**4**:158–62.

21 Anderson H, Hopwood P, Prendiville J, *et al*. A randomised study of intravenous bolus versus continuous pump infusion of ifosfamide and adriamycin with oral etoposide for "poor risk" small cell lung cancer. *Br J Cancer* 1993;**67**:1385–90.

22 Maguire P, Selby P. Assessing quality of life in cancer patients *Br J Cancer* 1989;**60**:437–40.

23 Zigmond AS, Snaith RD. The Hospital Anxiety and Depression Scale. *Acta Psychiatr Scand* 1983;**67**:361–70.

24 Fayers PM, Jones DR. Measuring and analysing quality of life in cancer clinical trials: A review. *Stat Med* 1983;**2**:429–46.

25 Fayers PM, Bleehen NM, Girling DJ, Stephens RJ. Assessment of quality of life in small cell lung cancer using a daily diary card developed by the Medical Research Council Lung Cancer Working Party. *Br J Cancer* 1991;**64**:299–306.

26 Geddes DM, Dones L, Hill E, Law K, Harper PG, Spiro SG. Quality of life during chemotherapy for small cell lung cancer: Assessment and use of a daily diary care in a randomised trial. *Eur J Cancer* 1990;**26**:484–92.

27 van Knippenberg FCE, de Haes JCJM. Measuring the quality of life of cancer patient: Psychometric properties of instruments. *J Clin Epidemiol* 1988;**41**:1043–53.

28 Goodwin PJ, Feld R, Evans WK, Pater J. Cost-effectiveness of cancer chemotherapy: An economic evaluation of a randomised trial in small-cell lung cancer. *J Clin Oncol* 1988;**6**:1537–47.

29 Goodwin PJ. Economic factors in cancer palliation—methodologic considerations. *Cancer Treat Rev* 1993;**19**(Suppl A): 59–65.

30 McVie JG. Counting costs of care. *Clin Oncol* 1988;**6**:1529–31.

31 Markman M. An argument in support of cost-effectiveness analysis in oncology. *J Clin Oncol* 1988;**6**:937–9.

32 Gelber RD, Goldhirsch A, Cole BF. Evaluation of effectiveness: Q-TWIST. *Cancer Treat Rev* 1993;**19**(Suppl A): 73–84.

33 Cox DR, Fitzpatrick R, Fletcher AE, Gore SM, Spiegelhalter DJ, Jones DR. Quality of life assessment: Can we keep it simple? *J R Statist Soc A* 1992;**155**:353–75.

34 Bakker W, van Oosterom AT, Aaronson NK, van Breukelan FJM, Bins MC, Hermans J. Vindesine, cisplatin and bleomycin combination chemotherapy in non-small cell lung cancer: survival and quality of life. *Br J Cancer Clin Oncol* 1986;**22**:963–70.

35 Cullen MH, Joshi R, Chetiyawardana AD, Woodroffe CM. Mitomycin, ifosfamide and cisplatin in non-small cell lung cancer: Treatment good enough to compare. *Br J Cancer* 1988;**58**:359–61.

36 Fernandez C, Rosell R, Abad-Esteve A, *et al*. Quality of life during chemotherapy in non-small cell lung cancer patients. *Acta Oncol* 1989;**28**:29–33.

37 Minet P, Bartsch P, Chevalier Ph, *et al*. Quality of life of inoperable non-small cell lung carcinoma: A randomised phase II clinical study comparing radiotherapy alone and combined radio-chemotherapy. *Radiother Oncol* 1987;**8**:271–80.

38 Thatcher N, Cerny T, Stout R, *et al*. Ifosfamide, etoposide and thoracic irradiation therapy in 163 patients with unresectable small cell lung cancer. *Cancer* 1987;**60**:1382–7.

39 Cella DF, Orofiamma B, Holland JC, *et al*. The relationship of psychological distress, extent of disease and performance status in patients with lung cancer. *Cancer* 1987;**60**:1661–7.

40 Mackillop WJ, Ward GK, O'Sullivan B. The use of expert surrogates to evaluate clinical trials in non-small cell lung cancer. *Br J Cancer* 1986;**54**:661–7.

41 Kaasa S, Mastekaasa A, Naess S. Quality of life of lung cancer patients in a randomized clinical trial evaluated by a psychosocial wellbeing questionnaire. *Acta Oncol* 1988;**27**:335–42.

42 Medical Research Council Lung Cancer Working Party. Inoperable non-small cell cancer (NSCLC): a Medical Research Council randomised trial of palliative radiotherapy with two fractions or ten fractions. *Br J Cancer* 1991;**63**:265–70.

43 Medical Research Council Lung Cancer Working Party. A Medical Research Council (MRC) randomised trial of palliative radiotherapy with two fractions or a single fraction in patients with inoperable non-small cell lung cancer (NSCLC) and a poor performance status. *Br J Cancer* 1992;**65**:934–41.

44 Silberfarb PM, Holland JCB, Anbar D, *et al.* Psychological response of patients receiving two drug regimens for lung carcinoma. *Am J Psychiatry* 1983;**140**:110–11.

45 Wolf M, Pritsch M, Drings P, *et al.* Cyclic-alternating versus response-orientated chemotherapy in small cell lung cancer: a German multicenter randomised trial of 321 patients. *J Clin Oncol* 1991;**9**:614–24.

46 Bergman B, Sullivan M, Sørenson S. Quality of life during chemotherapy for small cell lung cancer II. A longitudinal study of the EORTC Core Quality of Life Questionnaire and comparison with the Sickness Impact Profile. (MD Thesis) University of Goteborg, 1991.

47 Bleehen NM, Fayers PM, Girling DJ, Stephen RJ for British Medical Research Council Lung Cancer Working Party. Survival, adverse reactions and quality of life during combination chemotherapy compared with selective palliative treatment for small cell lung cancer. *Respir Med* 1989;**83**:51–8.

48 Bleehen NM, Fayers PM, Girling DJ, Stephens RJ. Contolled trial of twelve versus six courses of chemotherapy in the treatment of small cell lung cancer. *Br J Cancer* 1989;**59**:584–90.

49 Earl HM, Rudd RM, Spiro SG, *et al.* A randomised trial of planned versus as required chemotherapy in small lung cancer: a Cancer Research Campaign trial. *Br J Cancer* 1991;**64**:566–72.

50 British Medical Research Council Lung Cancer Working Party. Psychological distress as a component of quality of life (QOL) in a prospective randomised trials of two chemotherapy regimens for small cell lung cancer (SCLC). *Lung Cancer* 1991;**145**(Suppl7):540A.

51 Deyo RA, Patrick DL. Barriers to the use of Health Status Measures in clinical investigation, patient care and policy research. *Med Care* 1989;**27**:254–68.

52 Zwinderman AH. The measurement of change of quality of life in clinical trials. *Stat Med* 1990;**9**:931–42.

53 Osoba D. Self-rating symptom checklists: a simple method for recording and evaluating symptom control in oncology. *Cancer Treat Rev* 1993;**19**(Suppl A):43–51.

54 Spiegelhalter DJ, Gore SM, Fitzpatrick R, *et al.* Quality of life measures in health care: III. Resource Allocation. *BMJ* 1992;**305**:1205–9.

11 Patient benefit in clinical trials

MAURICE L SLEVIN, JEAN MOSSMAN

A large number of clinical trials have tested different therapeutic regimens for the treatment of lung cancer, but long term survival is still very poor.[1] Consequently, there is a degree of disillusionment with clinical trials for lung cancer, despite the recommendation from a Workshop on Consensus Guidelines for Management of Lung Cancer that, "All clinicians involved in the treatment of this disease should consider entering their patients into carefully controlled trials".[2] Clinical trials are generally accepted as the only reliable way to compare two or more treatment options (whether for a survival or palliative advantage, or difference to the quality of life), but the possible benefits for cancer patients who participate in clinical research are rarely considered.

The purpose of this chapter is to show that participation in clinical trials can benefit the individual with lung cancer, as well as increasing knowledge about the disease. It is intended to encourage clinicians to try to identify suitable clinical trials into which patients with lung cancer may be entered.

Why are trials needed?

Any treatment that has a major effect on the outcome of a disease will be readily identified. A randomised trial would be unnecessary in such circumstances. But the reality is that no such treatments for lung cancer have been found. Nevertheless, in a disease that kills one person every 13 minutes, even a small gain in survival would have a major impact. For example, a survival increase of 5% would save the lives of 2000 people each year in England and Wales alone, and since many of these deaths occur in middle age, prolonging these lives would clearly be worth while. Such small, but useful, treatment differences can only be identified with any certainty by assessing the effects in very large numbers of patients.

It would be reassuring to know that all treatments in current use have been "tried and tested", but this is not the case. Many standard treatments have never been subjected to rigorous evaluation. The limited resources available in the current financial climate have encouraged the Department of Health to examine the way in which new technologies are introduced. A Working Party from the Department has produced a report, which states that, "Randomised trials of sufficient size should be performed to . . . assess recently introduced technologies, the effects of which are unknown".[3] What is needed now is a new approach to ensure that sufficient numbers of patients are entered into trials within a reasonable time scale to answer important clinical questions.

What can trials show?

Treatment trials are recognised as being the optimal way to test whether a new treatment—or a novel combination of treatments—is better than the current standard treatment. But trials are more flexible than that. They are increasingly used to identify exactly which group of patients can be expected to benefit from the different treatment options available. They may show that the treatment tolerated by a young, fit patient is too demanding for an older or less fit patient, and they may show that the stage and grade of the disease might alter the response to treatment. The ability to identify with some precision which patients would benefit from a particular treatment would be a major advance in the management of any disease. Efforts have been made to use prognostic factors to try to identify long term survivors, and an overview of prognostic factors from several United Kingdom trials of small cell lung cancer was undertaken in 1990 by the United Kingdom Coordinating Committee on Cancer Research (UKCCCR) Lung Subcommittee.[4] This recommended that performance status, disease stage, alkaline phosphatase, sodium, aspartate aminotransferase, and lactate dehydrogenase should be measured in all future studies of small cell lung cancer, and that this could assist in the selection of patients for different treatment strategies. This overview is to be updated in 1993 by the Medical Research Council (MRC). Trials may identify whether two treatments have a cumulative effect, or whether the different treatments interact. They may also show whether treatment in specialist centres confers an advantage.[5] External factors may mediate—for example, when only limited resources and facilities are available locally: trials can be designed to accommodate these local differences.

The MRC has looked at practical questions in some of its trials, and shown that radiotherapy, which is the most effective treatment for local, intrathoracic symptoms, is as effective when given by 17 Gy in two fractions as 30 Gy given in 10 fractions.[6] It has subsequently shown that one fraction is as effective as two in poor risk patients.[7] These results have important implications both for the provision of radiotherapy services and for the convenience of patients, who need only attend once rather than 10 times to achieve the same degree of palliation.

The question of an absolute survival benefit is not the only factor which patients consider when deciding whether to undergo treatment. If, as in lung cancer, the expected benefit is small, the issues of convenience, quality of life, and cost all have a role in the equation. If an unpleasant treatment requires a lengthy round trip to receive it the patient might not consider the probable small benefit worth while. If the patient's remaining time is likely to be uncomfortable or complicated by harrowing treatment this may be more than the patient is prepared to accept. In assessing the value of trials in palliative chemotherapy—which, in lung cancer, is the realistic role of cytotoxic treatment in most patients—a measure of quality of life is therefore essential. Quality of life measures make it possible to determine benefit from the patient's point of view, regardless of objective toxicity, and to distinguish the best regimen from two otherwise identical treatments. Several studies using quality of life measures have produced unexpected results, with patients preferring the more toxic treatment because the improved responses have had quality of life benefits.[8 9]

The MRC has looked at the question of quality of life after chemotherapy in patients with small cell lung cancer. The gain from chemotherapy is modest because few patients achieve long term survival, so the quality of life during and after treatment assumes even greater importance. The MRC found that although maintenance chemotherapy adversely affects quality of life, this concerns only the first two or three days following each course of treatment; patients allocated no maintenance treatment experienced a gradually deteriorating quality of life.[10]

How does an individual patient gain?

There is some evidence to suggest that patients fare better when treated in the context of a treatment trial; there is certainly no evidence that inclusion in properly conducted trials results in poorer survival. Little formal research has been carried out on this in the context of adult cancers, but a substantial amount of research on the outcome of childhood leukaemias has been undertaken.[11]

How does taking part in a clinical trial benefit the patient? What are the potential advantages of being treated on a research protocol? One advantage of treatment trials is that the protocol has been very carefully worked out by experts in the field to ensure that the novel approach to be tested is being compared with the best available treatment. Only by comparing new treatments with gold standards can their real benefit be properly assessed. Considerable effort will have been put into ensuring that only patients suitable for either treatment will be entered, and that the treatments being proposed (and supportive measures, if important) are accurately described so that mistakes are less likely. The protocol will have been examined by a local research ethics committee to ensure that sick patients are not being treated improperly. Patients are likely to be given more information about their type of cancer, and will have access to medical staff experienced in treating the disease. Patients in trials are often treated in specialist centres where, because the clinicians have a particular interest in the disease, there are usually good facilities for the supportive care that is important in avoiding or alleviating suffering. Patients may also undergo more tests and investigations as part of a trial, but this is increasingly being limited to phase I and II trials where smaller numbers of patients are needed.

What do patients think?

A recent survey undertaken by the UKCCCR of 75 patients being treated for a variety of cancers in eight oncology units asked how they viewed clinical research. The patients were aged between 17 and 83 (mean age 50·1 years), and 48% of them were males.

Most patients were being seen by medical oncologists, and for 76% it was their first visit to that particular clinic. Most had been referred by another specialist, but about one third had been referred directly from their general practitioner.

Patients were asked which aspects of clinical trials they found greatly or slightly appealing, and greatly or slightly unappealing (table I). Responses indicated that most patients were attracted to the idea that progress was monitored closely, that there was a greater chance of being treated by a doctor with a specialist interest in the disease, that taking part contributed to research knowledge and benefited humanity, and that being in a trial meant that they would be likely to obtain more information about their condition. After being asked to rank 10 items patients were asked to identify the three most important. The results of this choice showed that being looked after by a specialist was regarded by 36% of patients as being the most important aspect of clinical trials. Being given a chance to use new treatments and contributing to research knowledge and benefiting humanity were the other two aspects which most patients rated as important.

Respondents were asked if they thought they would agree to take part in a research trial for their illness. It was explained that, "this would mean that you would be allocated to *either* the new treatment *or* to standard treatments". Perhaps unexpectedly, as few as 10% of patients indicated that they would not be willing to take part in clinical trials. The others were either willing (42%) or uncertain (48%). Those who replied that they would not agree to take part or were uncertain were asked why. The respondents were

Table I   Items patients were asked to rank as greatly or slightly appealing, and greatly or slightly unappealing

1	Treatment decided by doctor
2	More tests/investigations carried out
3	Contributes to research knowledge and benefits humanity
4	More likely to be treated by doctors with special interest in your type of cancer
5	Greater chance of obtaining new treatments
6	Treatments more likely to be decided by panel of experts
7	Progress monitored closely
8	Likely to obtain more information about condition
9	Greater chance of obtaining experimental treatments
10	Don't choose treatment oneself

most likely to select as their reason "would prefer doctor to make the decision about the treatment" (51%), and "would worry about receiving new treatment" (33%); 9% selected "would prefer to be able to choose treatment".

This study suggested that most patients are either enthusiastic or uncertain about entering clinical trials. Only a small percentage are unwilling to participate. The most difficult aspect for patients to grasp is the issue of randomisation—having their treatment selected by computer. More widespread knowledge about trials would mean that these sorts of concepts could be dealt with when patients were more receptive, and there is much to be said for general practitioners explaining the concept of randomisation to patients when they advise them that they need to be referred for a specialist opinion.

Health economics

The recent publication from the Department of Health, *Assessing the Effects of Health Technologies*, emphasises the importance of clinical trials for identifying which new treatments are an improvement over conventional ones, and states that where the optimal treatment is unknown, patients should be treated within trials.[3] This recommendation is partly an attempt to ensure that new treatments are not introduced in an uncontrolled way, and partly an attempt to ensure that the implications for the NHS are investigated alongside the assessment of the efficacy of the novel treatment or regimen. At present too little information is available about the true benefits and costs of different treatment approaches. Many clinicians believe that they can calculate the cost of a treatment quite simply by obtaining the cost of the drugs administered and multiplying this figure by the number of courses, and adding on the cost of a short hospital stay or an outpatient visit. The reality is different. One treatment may improve quality of life to a much greater degree than another; one treatment may require much more in the way of supportive care than another; one treatment may have long term sequelae that result in the patient attending outpatient clinics or general practitioner surgeries for an extended period.

Unless the real costs of treatments can be calculated it is impossible to plan the proper provision of health care facilities. Trials are now addressing these sorts of issues more realistically.

Perhaps more importantly to the individual patient, such assessments also include the benefit to the patients in terms of survival and quality of life, and the cost to the patient—in actual costs, or inconvenience, or time away from work or home. This information is an essential prerequisite to allow properly informed choices about treatments to be made. Issues on health economics have to be included in trial design so that not only the questions "Is there a benefit?" and "What size is the benefit?" are addressed, but also "At what cost to the patient and his or her family?". These issues are currently being examined as a major part of the Continuous Hyperfractionated Accelerated Radiotherapy Trial (CHART) being conducted by the Cancer Research Campaign, the Department of Health, and the MRC.

There is, of course, a cost to the doctor of participating in trials. At present there is a disincentive for doctors to enter patients into clinical trials because of the extra work involved and very little associated benefit. Urgent consideration must be given by the Department of Health to supporting their stated position by providing incentives to encourage doctors to undertake this extra work.

How to identify a trial for your patients

Most major oncology departments have treatment trials in progress, and the first step in identifying a suitable trial is to seek advice from the appropriate specialist. The MRC runs a national programme of trials which draws participants from many of the district general hospitals across the country, so that patients do not have to travel long distances to take part. The Cancer Research Campaign also has a programme of multicentre trials. Other groups run trials, often on a multicentre basis, but perhaps confined to one or two regions or districts. There is a register of ongoing treatment trials in cancer, compiled by the UKCCCR and maintained as an on-line database at the MRC Cancer Trials Office in Cambridge. This can be accessed to identify trials suitable for each patient. There might be no suitable trials, but if demand for trials can be achieved resources are likely to be provided to set up trials to address important health questions.

Lung cancer is an important health problem, but as a result of the lack of enthusiasm for trials by the broad range of clinicians treating the disease only a limited number of trials have been set up, and only a tiny proportion of patients are being entered into these. It is time that this changed, and that patients are given the opportunity to receive the best possible treatment—and where this is not known, to take part in trials in order to define the best treatment.

The telephone number of the MRC Trials Office in Cambridge is 0223 311110.

1 Souhami RL, Law K. Longevity in small cell lung cancer. *Br J Cancer* 1990;**61**:584–9.
2 Timothy AR. Consensus Statement. Workshop on Consensus Guidelines for Management of Lung Cancer. *Clin Oncol* 1990;**2**:97–101.
3 Advisory Group for Health Technology Assessment. *Assessing the effects of health technologies*. Department of Health Research and Development Directorate. London: DOH/HMSO, 1992.
4 Rawson NSB, Peto J. An overview of prognostic factors in small cell lung cancer. A report from the Subcommittee for the Management of Lung Cancer of the United Kingdom Coordinating Committee on Cancer Research. *Br J Cancer* 1990;**61**:597–604.
5 Harding MJ, Paul J, Gillis R, Keye SB. Management of malignant teratoma: does referral to a specialist unit matter? *Lancet* 1993;**341**:999–1002.
6 Medical Research Council Lung Cancer Working Party. Inoperable non-small cell lung cancer (NSCLC): a Medical Research Council randomised trial of palliative radiotherapy with two fractions or ten fractions. *Br J Cancer* 1991;**63**:265–70.
7 A Medical Research Council (MRC) randomised trial of palliative radiotherapy with 2 fractions or a single fraction in patients with inoperable non-small cell lung cancer (NSCLC) and a poor performance status. *Br J Cancer* 1992;**65**:934–41.
8 Slevin ML. Quality of life: philosophical question or clinical reality? *BMJ* 1992;**305**:466–9.
9 Kaasa S, Mastekaasa A, Naess S. Quality of life of lung cancer patients in a randomized clinical trial evaluated by a psychosocial well-being questionnaire. *Acta Oncol* 1988;**27**:335–42.
10 Fayers PM, Bleehen NM, Girling DJ, Stephens RJ. Assessment of quality of life in small-cell lung cancer using a Daily Diary Card developed by the Medical Research Council Lung Cancer Working Party. *Br J Cancer* 1991;**64**:299–306.
11 Stiller C. Survival of patients in clinical trials and at specialist centres. In: Williams CS, ed. *Introducing new treatments for cancer*. 1992:19–36.

Index

Drug combinations are indexed by individual drugs

abdomen
  computed tomograms 92
  metastases 89
adenocarcinoma 23, 26, 34, 42,
  69, 151
adrenal glands 92
adrenocorticotrophic hormone 38
age of patients 79
AIDS 127
airway epithelium 30–31
albumin 98, 156
alkaline phosphatase 80, 98, 108,
  130
alveolar cell carcinoma 20
amines 31, 38
anaemia 123
androgens 58–59
angina 93
angiotensin 53
anorexia 113
antigen workshops 73
antigens 68
  binding to extracellular matrix
    proteins 71
  blood group 73
  carcinoembryonic 69–70
  classification 73, 74
  clinical approaches 74-76
  transmembrane signal induction
    73
anxiety 165, 171
appetite 156
aspartate aminotransferase 98,
  108
autocrine growth
  stimulation 51–52, 60, 72
  control 154–155

azatoxin 149

benzene 15
benzo(a)pyrene – DNA
  adducts 22
bilirubin 80
Blackman, Lionel 14
bladder cancer 21, 125
blood group antigens 73
blood progenitor cells 134–135,
  137
blood tests 80
biopsy 36, 81
  percutaneous needle 84
  transbronchial 84
bombesin analogues 61
bombesin/gastrin releasing
  peptide 52–55
  receptor 53, 62
  signalling pathways 53–55
bone marrow
  cells 122, 138, 139
  examination 97
  suppression 124, 134, 138
  transplantation 127, 133–134
bone metastases 92, 96
bone pain 129, 130
bradykinin 53, 57
brain metastases 92, 96
  prophylactic cranial irradiation
    171–172
brain scans 92, 96
breast cancer 22, 25, 60, 133
breathlessness 113
British-American Tobacco
  Industries Ltd 14

British Code of Advertising
    Practice 12
bronchial dysplasia 24
bronchial obstruction 117
bronchial washes 81
bronchodilation 95
brnchoscopy 80–81
bryostatin 62
busulphan 133

C-*fos* genes 54
C-*jun* genes 47
C-*myc* genes 54, 155
C reactive protein 80
cachexia 156
calcitonin 38
calcium 80
    mobilisation 53, 54, 56, 57, 59
calcium channel blockers 62
camptothecin analogues 146–147,
    151
Canada 11, 173
    National Cancer Institute 148
Cancer Research Campaign 183
carbohydrate antigens 73
carboplatin 124, 132, 144,
    149–150, 152
carcinoembryonic antigens 69–70,
    80
carcinogens
    cigarette smoke 3, 15, 22, 25
    metabolism 21–22
carcinoid tumours 36
    atypical 32, 39–42
    classification 32, 33, 34, 35
    diagnosis and prognosis 38–39
    histology 37–39
    metastases 39
    paragangloid 38
cardiac symptoms 95
cardiothoracic surgeon 89
carmustine 133
cell 68
    cycle 138
    growth factor production 122
    membrane receptors 71–73
    signal pathways 53–55
cell-cell attachment
    molecules 69–71

Centre for Health Economics 172
cervical cancer 25
CHART protocol 111, 113, 183
chemotherapy 99–100, 179–180
    accelerated 131–133
    advanced lung cancer 106–111,
    117
    duration 108–109
    haematopoietic growth factors
    123, 124–135, 139
    non-small cell cancer 94, 117,
    126–127, 150–154
    new drugs 146–150
    quality of life 107, 111, 156,
    170, 171, 179–180
    when to assess new
      drugs 144–146
chest pain 95, 113
chest radiography 79–80, 84
chest symptoms 95, 113
child smoking 5, 8–10
    predictors 12
    prevention 14–15
cholecystokinin 56–57
cholesterol 130
chromogranin A 32, 44, 47
chromosomes 23
    deletions 24
    3p site 24, 25, 47
cigarette smoke
    carcinogens 3, 15
    environmental 7
cigarette smoking 2
    children and young people 5–6,
    8–10, 12, 14–15
    genetics 19, 20
    passive 6–7
    personal reasons 7–10
    prevalence 3, 4, 5
    prevention 13–15
    risk of lung cancer 6
    state or government 10–13
    trends 4–6
cigarettes
    advertising 12–13
    availability 10
    consumption 4–5
    price 11

cigars 4, 12
cisplatin 123, 125, 128, 131, 133, 138, 144, 145
clinical trials
  chemotherapy 106–111, 117
  cost/benefit 182–183
  identifying 183–184
  immunotherapy 117
  non-small cell lung cancer 111–118, 152
  patient benefit 105, 177–183
  radiotherapy 111–117
  small cell lung cancer 106–111, 147
  views of patients 180–182
cobalt miners 2
collagen 71
Committee for Monitoring Agreements on Tobacco Advertising and Sponsorship (COMATAS) 12
computed tomograms 82, 86, 89, 92
  sensitivity/specificity 91
cost/benefit 182–183
cost effectiveness/quality of life 166–167
  trial 172
costs See financial costs
cough 113
CPT-11 147, 152
Cushing's syndrome 31
cyclophosphamide 106, 108, 109, 125, 129, 131, 133, 134, 136, 138, 145, 146, 149
cystitis, haemorrhagic 148, 149
cytology 81
cytopenia 127

debrisoquine 21
dehydrotestosterone 58
dense core neurosecretory granules 37–38, 41, 42–43, 46
4′-deoxydoxorubicin 152
Department of Health 5, 178, 183
  Assessing the Effects of Health Technologies 182
depression 165, 171
1, 2-diacylglycerol 53–54

diagnosis
  carcinoid tumours 38–39
  history, examination and chest radiograph 79–80
  investigation pathway 78
  neuroendocrine tumours 35–36
  peripheral mass lesion 82–84
  precise 79
  thoracic computed tomograms 82
diary card See patient diary card
diffuse neuroendocrine system 31
DNA 148
  analysis 24
  damage 21, 25
  mutatin 21, 25
  polymorphisms 23
  repair enzymes 22
  technology 122
doxorubicin 109, 124, 125, 129, 131, 136, 145, 146,
dysphagia 95, 113, 115

Eastern Cooperative Oncology Group 146
echocardiography 95
ecogenetics 21–22
10-EDAM 152, 153
electron microscopy 35, 36
emesis 156
endobronchial treatment 95, 117
endocrine tumours, atypical 34
endothelial cells 122
endothelins 53
environment
  genetic susceptibility 21
  tobacco smoke 7
eosinophilia 127
eosinophils 122, 127, 128, 129
epidemiological studies 20
epidermal growth factor receptor 60, 61, 71–72
epipodophyllotoxins 148–149
epirubicin 147, 148, 152
erythrocytes 120, 122
erythropoietin 122, 123–124
ethyol WR2721 138
etoposide 108, 109, 111, 144, 145, 149

etoposide—*contd*
  haematopoietic growth factor
    use 124, 125, 128, 129, 131,
    132, 133, 136, 138
European Communities 11
European Organisation for
  Research and Treatment of
  Cancer (EORTC)
  quality of life questionnaire 164
  trials 108, 150
exercise tolerance 93
extracellular matrix 71

FACT scale 164, 166
familial clustering 20–21
fetal lung 52
FEV1/FVC 93
fibreoptic bronchoscopy 80
  complications,
    contraindications,
    mortality 81
fibroblasts 122
films 12
financial costs 82, 91, 92, 93,
  135–136
fotemustine 152–153
Functional Assessment of Cancer
  Therapy 164, 166
Functional Living Index – Cancer
  163

G proteins 53
galanin 57
gastrin 56–57
gastrin releasing peptide 38, 44,
  52, 56
gemcitabine 152, 153
General Household Surveys 5
genetic changes 155
  cytogenetic analysis 23
  deletion and allele loss 24–26
  molecular studies 23–24
  mutations and amplification 26
genetic predisposition 19–23
  epidemiological studies 20
  environment 21–22
  familial clustering 20–21
  linkage studies 22–23
  smoking 19, 20
glutathione transferase 22

(glycolate-0,0') diammineplatinum
  (II) 152
glycolipid antigens 71, 73
glycoproteins
  gp 40 70, 73
  p 72 72
  myelin associated 70
government 10–13
  prevention of smoking 13–15
granulocyte colony stimulating
  factor 59, 122, 137, 138
  clinical use 124–127, 131–135
  cost 135–136
  pharmacology 128–130
  side effects 130–131
granulocyte macrophage colony
  stimulating factor 59, 122,
  127–128, 131–135, 137, 138
  cost 135–136
  pharmacology 128–129
  toxicity 128, 130
granulocytes 120, 122, 127
granulocytopenia 151
growth factors
  non-small cell cancer 60
  small cell cancer 44–45, 51–60
  therapeutic implications 60–62
  see also haematopoietic growth
    factors

haematopoiesis 120
  inhibitors 139
haematopoietic growth factors 59,
  120–122, 155–156
  cell cycle 138
  clinical applications 122–135
  combinations 138
  cost considerations 135–137
  future 137–139
haemoglobin 80, 123
haemoptysis 113
health care expenditure 3–4
health economics 182–183
  cost of treatments 82, 91, 92,
    93, 135–136
  quality of life 166–167
health education 14
Health Education Authority 14
Health of the Nation 15

hilar nodes 89
historical review 1–2
HLA 71
hoarseness 95
Hospital Anxiety and Depression
    Scale 96, 111, 165, 171
hydrazine sulphate 156
5-hydroxy-tryptamine 38, 46
hypernephroma 84
hyponatraemia 56, 80

idarubicin 145
ifosfamide 109, 124, 129, 131,
    132, 138, 147, 149, 150
immunotherapy 117
infections, neutropenic 124, 126,
    127–128, 131, 132
inositol 1,4,5-triphosphate 53
Institut Gustave Roussy 117
Istituto Mario Negri 117
insulin-like growth factor I 58,
    154
    receptors 72
integrins 71
interferons 59, 62, 150
interleukins 122, 138, 156
    interleukin 2 147, 150, 152, 154
    interleukin 3 122, 137, 138
International Association for the
    Study of Lung Cancer 43
investigations
    chest symptoms 95
    diagnosis 77–87
    management 87–100
iododoxorubicin 152

K-ras gene 26
Karnofsky Index 98
    SCORES 68
Kulschitsky cells 31
    carcinoma 32, 35

lactate dehydrogenase 98, 108,
    131
laminin 71
large cell cancer 82
    classification 32–33
large cell neuroendocrine
    carcinomas 34, 41, 46

leu-enkephalin 38, 47
leucocytes 127, 129, 130
leucocytosis 127, 128, 130
Li-Fraumeni syndrome 20–21
light microscopy 35–36
Linear Analogue Self Assessment
    Scales 163
liposarcoma 127
liver metastases 92
lobectomy 93
London Lung Cancer Group 109
lonidamine 152
lung
    fetal 52
    function 93
    neuroendocrine cells 30–31
lung cancer
    development of histological
        types 68
    in the nineteenth century 1–2
    incidence 1
    mortality 1, 2–3, 143
    survival 143
lymph node histology 89–91
lymphangitis carcinomatosa 82
lymphocytes 122
lymphoma 84, 86

macrophages 122, 129
magazine advertising 12–13
magnetic resonance imaging 86
malignant melanoma 22, 133
    cells 70
management
    inoperable patients 93–94
    non-curative treatment 94–96
    non-small cell cancer 87–96
    small cell cancer 97–100
mediastinal lymph nodes 89, 91,
    92
    sampling 91, 93
mediastinum 89
    invasion 89
    masses 86
    symptoms 95
Medical Outcome Study Short
    Form General Health
    Survey 163
medroxyprogesterone acetate 156

megakaryocytes 124, 137
megakaryocytic colony stimulating factor 137
melanoma *See* malignant melanoma
melphalan 126
menogaril 146, 147
mesothelioma 84, 86, 138
metastases 98–99
    carcinoid tumours 39
    investigations 89, 96
    preoperative scanning 91–93
methotrexate 108, 109, 125
    analogue 153
Midlands Small Cell Lung Cancer Group 109
migration inhibitory antibody 80
mitozantrone 145
mitoxolomide 147
mixed small cell/large cell carcinoma 43
molecular biology 23–24, 255
monoclonal antibodies 74–76
    antigen workshops 73, 74
    bombesin 61
monocytes 122, 128
mouse genetics 22
MRC Cancer Therapy Committee 165
MRC Cancer Trials Office 117, 173
    address 118
    database 183
    telephone number 184
MRC Lung Cancer Working Party 106, 113, 115, 116, 117, 136
    quality of life 165, 171
MRC trials 108, 109, 110, 111, 179, 183
    quality of life/cost effectiveness trial 172
mucins 73
myc genes 26, 47, 54
myelin associated glycoprotein 70
myelodysplastic syndromes 127

naloxone 58
navelbine 147, 151, 152

neural cell adhesion molecule (NCAM) 32, 47, 69
    isoforms 70
    monoclonal antibodies 73
neuroendocrine differentiation
    carcinoid tumours 36–42
    cells 30–31
    diagnostic difficulties 35–36
    lung tumour classification 31–35
    markers 32, 36, 46–47
    non-small cell carcinoma 45–46
    small cell carcinoma 42–45
neurofibromatosis 22
neuromedin B 56
neurone specific enolase 32, 44, 46, 80
neuropathy 151
neuropeptides 51, 52, 53, 55
neurotensin 57
neutropenia 124, 125, 129, 132, 135
    febrile 126, 128, 136
neutrophils 122, 124, 126, 128, 129, 133, 135
nidogen 71
nifedipine 62
non-small cell cancer
    chemotherapy 94, 117, 118, 126–127, 150–154
    endobronchial treatment 117
    genetics 21, 25
    growth factors 60
    immunotherapy 117
    inoperable 93–96, 113
    neuroendocrine differentiation 34, 45–46
    quality of life trial 172
    radiotherapy 94, 95, 111–116
    surgery 87–93
    survival 95, 143–144
Northern Ireland 3–4

oat cell carcinoma 42
oncogenes 26, 155
opioids 57–58
ovarian cancer 22, 138

p53 gene 21, 25, 47

p185^{neu} 60
Pancoast tumour 86
paragangliomas 38
paraneoplastic syndromes 45
    presentations 96
Parents against Tobacco 10
passive smoking 6–7
patient diary card 107, 111, 112,
    165–166
    compliance 170
patients
    average age 79
    compliance 170, 171
    questionnaires 163
    views 180–182
peptides 31, 51
    antagonists 61
    secretion 31–32, 38, 44, 55
percutaneous needle biopsy 84
performance status 98, 108
peripheral masses 81, 82
    investigation pathway 83
    percutaneous needle biopsy 84
Perrier water 15
PGP 9.5 32, 46
phosphohexose isomerase 80
physalaemin 59
pipe smoking 4
pirarubicin 147, 148–149, 152
platelet derived growth factor 72
platelets 122, 127, 130
platinum drugs 150–151, 153
pleural disease 85–86, 95
pneumonectomy 93
polyerase chain reaction 24
progenitor cells 134–135, 137
prophylactic cranial irradiation
    171–172
Protection of Young People
    (Tobacco) Bill 10
protein kinase C 54
protocols 118
    CHART 111, 113, 183
    LU16 111
    LU17 116
    LU18 117
    LU20 118
psychological symptoms 96

Quality added life years (QALYS)
    173–174
quality of life 107–108, 111, 156,
    161, 179–180
    assessment 162–166, 167–171
    bibliographic and index 163
    cost effectiveness 166–167, 172
    defining 162
    proxy measures 167–168
    research 171–174
questionnaires 163

radiation myelopathy 113, 115
radiotherapy 179
    CHART 111, 113, 172, 183
    external beam 95, 117
    palliative 94, 95, 113–116
    prophylactic 171–172
    radical 111–113
ras oncogenes 47
referral and start of treatment 96
renal cancer 25
renal failure 123, 153
restriction fragment length
    polymorphisms 23
retail price index 11
reticulocytes 127, 130
retinoblastoma gene 21, 25, 26, 47
RFLP analysis 24
Rotterdam Symptom Checklist
    111, 164–165, 171
Royal College of Physicians 4

Scotland 1
serotonin 53
Sickness Impact Profile 163
signal pathways 53–55
skin masses 86
small cell cancer
    bombesin/gastrin releasing
        peptide 52–55
    classification 32, 33, 34, 42
    genetics 21, 23, 24, 25, 26
    growth factors synthesised 51,
        55
    growth inhibiting factors 59–60
    growth stimulation 56–59
    prognosis and staging 97–100,
        108, 178

small cell cancer—*contd*
    survival 99, 106, 143
    tumour marker 80
    See also chemotherapy
smoking *See* cigarette smoking
soap operas 12
socioeconomic status 5
sodium 80, 98
somatostatin 38, 59
    analogues 60, 62
somatuline 60
South West Oncology Group 128
specialist centres 179
spirometry 93
sports sponsorship 12
sputum cytology 81
squamous cell carcinoma 20, 24,
    42, 71, 89, 151
stem cell factor 59
stromal cells 122
substance K 53
substance P 53
superior sulcus tumour 86
superior vena cava obstruction 95
supraventricular nodes 86
surgery
    assessment of operability 87–91
    fitness for 93
    preoperative scanning 91–93
Swiss 3T3 cells 52, 53, 54, 56, 57
synaptophysin 32, 47

tax increases 11
taxol 152
TCNU 152, 154
teenage smoking 5–6, 9–10
    reducing 14–15
tenascin 71
teniposide 144, 147, 149, 152
testosterone 58
thoracotomy
    cost of prevention 92
    futile 91
thrombocytopenia 128, 129, 132,
    138
thrombopoietin 138
thymoma 86
tobacco
    advertising 12

health care expenditure 4
industry 3, 11, 13, 14
taxes 11
Tobacco Advisory Council 5
topoisomerase inhibition 148, 149
topotecan (SKF104864) 148
tracheal obstruction 117
transbronchial fine needle
    aspiration 81, 84
transferrin 58
transforming growth factor α 60
transmembrane signal induction
    71–72
triglycidylurazole 145
trimetrexate 152, 153
tuberculosis 86
tumour classification 31–35, 42
tumour markers 32, 36, 44, 80
    neuroendocrine 46–47
tumour necrosis factor α 152, 154
tumour suppressor genes 22, 24,
    25, 47, 155
tyrosine phosphorylation 54

ultrasound scanning 85, 86, 89
United Kingdom Coordinating
    Committee on Cancer
    Research (UKCCCR) 171,
    178, 180
    register of trials 183
United States of America 11, 12,
    14, 173
    National Cancer Institute 60
uric acid 130

vasoactive intestinal polypeptide
    38, 53
vasopressin 53, 56
verapamil 62
"victim blaming" 10
vinblastine 125
vincristine 108, 109, 111, 131,
    145, 146
von Hippel-Lindau gene locus 24

women
    cigarette consumption 5

mortality 1, 3
smoking prevalence 5
World Health Organisation 98
lung tumour classification 32, 42

Yorkshire Cancer Registry 79, 88, 94, 96

zeniplatin 152, 153
zidovudine 127